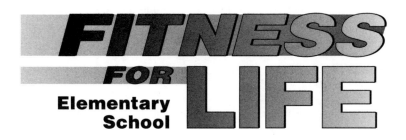

Elementary
School

# Classroom Guide
## SECOND GRADE

**Dolly D. Lambdin**

**Charles B. Corbin**

**Guy C. Le Masurier**

**Meg Greiner**

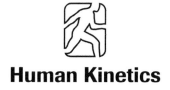

**Human Kinetics**

**Library of Congress Cataloging-in-Publication Data**

Fitness for life : elementary school classroom guide. Second grade / Dolly D. Lambdin ... [et al.].
   p. cm.
 Includes bibliographical references.
 ISBN-13: 978-0-7360-8602-8 (soft cover)
 ISBN-10: 0-7360-8602-1 (soft cover)
 1.  Physical fitness for children--Study and teaching (Elementary)  I. Lambdin, Dolly, 1951-
 GV443.F5255 2010
 372.86--dc22

                2009047175

ISBN-10: 0-7360-8602-1 (print)
ISBN-13: 978-0-7360-8602-8 (print)

The Web addresses cited in this text were current as of December 2009, unless otherwise noted.

**Acquisitions Editor:** Scott Wikgren; **Developmental Editor:** Ray Vallese; **Assistant Editor:** Derek Campbell; **Copyeditor:** Mary Rivers; **Permission Manager:** Dalene Reeder; **Graphic Designer:** Fred Starbird; **Graphic Artist:** Denise Lowry; **Cover Designer:** Keith Blomberg; **Photographer (cover):** © Human Kinetics; **Photographer (interior):** © Human Kinetics, unless otherwise specified; lower photo on p. 1 © Monika Adamczyk/fotolia.com; lower photo on p. 21 © Comstock; photos on pp. 15, 39, 113, and 128 by Neil Bernstein; **Photo Asset Manager:** Laura Fitch; **Visual Production Assistant:** Joyce Brumfield; **Photo Production Manager:** Jason Allen; **Art Manager:** Kelly Hendren; **Associate Art Manager:** Alan L. Wilborn; **Illustrator:** Keri Evans, unless otherwise specified; **Printer:** Versa Press

Printed in the United States of America    10  9  8  7  6  5  4  3  2  1

The paper in this book is certified under a sustainable forestry program.

**Human Kinetics**
Web site: www.HumanKinetics.com

*United States:* Human Kinetics, P.O. Box 5076, Champaign, IL 61825-5076
800-747-4457
e-mail: humank@hkusa.com

*Canada:* Human Kinetics, 475 Devonshire Road Unit 100, Windsor, ON N8Y 2L5
800-465-7301 (in Canada only)
e-mail: info@hkcanada.com

*Europe:* Human Kinetics, 107 Bradford Road, Stanningley, Leeds LS28 6AT, United Kingdom
+44 (0) 113 255 5665
e-mail: hk@hkeurope.com

*Australia:* Human Kinetics, 57A Price Avenue, Lower Mitcham, South Australia 5062
08 8372 0999
e-mail: info@hkaustralia.com

*New Zealand:* Human Kinetics, P.O. Box 80, Torrens Park, South Australia, 5062
0800 222 062
e-mail: info@hknewzealand.com

E4906

# CONTENTS

## PART I

## GETTING STARTED
## 1

## PART II

## LESSON PLANS
## 21

# LESSON FINDER

· · · · · · · · · · · · · · · · · · · · · · · · · · · · · ·

This guide provides 20 lesson plans—one plan for each day of the four Wellness Weeks that will be conducted throughout the school year. This Lesson Finder will help you easily locate each of the lesson plans as you conduct the activities throughout the year.

| Week | Day | Morning Activity Break | Special Day Activities | Afternoon Activity Break |
|------|-----|------------------------|------------------------|--------------------------|
| 1 | 1<br>page 27 | Get Fit<br>Message: Be active every day. | — | Head, Shoulders, Knees, and Toes |
| | 2<br>page 32 | Get Fit<br>Message: Keep on trying. | — | Pattern Practice |
| | 3<br>page 36 | Get Fit<br>Message: Fitness foods | Eat Well Wednesday:<br>• Discussion: Track Your Fruits and Veggies<br>• Activity: A to Z Fruit and Veggie Bar in the Cafeteria | Simon Says |
| | 4<br>page 42 | Get Fit<br>Message: Play safely. | — | Follow the Leader |
| | 5<br>page 46 | Get Fit<br>Message: I can, you can, we all can. | Get Fit Friday:<br>TEAM Time 1: School Walk | Alphabet Lineup |
| 2 | 1<br>page 55 | La Raspa<br>Message: Get your body moving. | — | Itsy Bitsy Spider |
| | 2<br>page 60 | La Raspa<br>Message: Get better with practice. | — | Pattern Practice |
| | 3<br>page 64 | La Raspa<br>Message: Foods with fats (discussions also feature grains) | Eat Well Wednesday:<br>• Discussion: Whole Grains and Breakfast<br>• Activity: Healthy Breakfast Promotion | Simon Says |
| | 4<br>page 70 | La Raspa<br>Message: Exercise your heart. | — | Follow the Leader |
| | 5<br>page 74 | La Raspa<br>Message: Never, ever give up! | Get Fit Friday:<br>TEAM Time 2: Big Kids Lead | Shirt Color Lineup |

| Week | Day | Morning Activity Break | Special Day Activities | Afternoon Activity Break |
|------|-----|------------------------|------------------------|--------------------------|
| **3** | **1**<br>page 83 | Wave It<br>Message: Get your muscles ready. | — | If You're Happy and You Know It |
| | **2**<br>page 88 | Wave It<br>Message: Move your body. | — | Pattern Practice |
| | **3**<br>page 92 | Wave It<br>Message: Food for strong bones and muscles | Eat Well Wednesday:<br>• Discussion: Fuel Up: Foods With Protein<br>• Activity: Fuel Up: Yogurt Bar in the Cafeteria | Simon Says |
| | **4**<br>page 98 | Wave It<br>Message: You have only one body; make it fit! | — | Follow the Leader |
| | **5**<br>page 102 | Wave It<br>Message: If it is to be, it's up to me. | Get Fit Friday:<br>TEAM Time 3: Little Kids Lead | Shoe Color Lineup |
| **4** | **1**<br>page 111 | It's the One<br>Message: Get off your seat and move your feet. | — | Alphabet Song |
| | **2**<br>page 116 | It's the One<br>Message: Play lots, learn lots. | — | Pattern Practice |
| | **3**<br>page 120 | It's the One<br>Message: Healthy food helps us move. | Eat Well Wednesday:<br>• Discussion: Eat Fat Sparingly; Avoid Empty Calories<br>• Activity: Fruit and Veggie Bar With Bottled Water in the Cafeteria | Simon Says |
| | **4**<br>page 126 | It's the One<br>Message: Be water wise. | — | Follow the Leader |
| | **5**<br>page 130 | It's the One<br>Message: Plan to get better. | Get Fit Friday:<br>TEAM Time 4: Mid Kids Lead | Birthday Lineup |

# PREFACE

**Fitness for Life: Elementary School** is a unique program that focuses attention on schoolwide wellness during four weeks of the school year. A primary objective of the program is to help schools incorporate coordinated activities that will enable them to meet national standards and guidelines for physical activity and nutrition as part of their school wellness policy. The program promotes healthy lifestyles in physical education and classrooms as well as in the entire school and community. Featured components of healthy lifestyles are sound nutrition and regular physical activity. The program is designed specifically for elementary school students and provides lesson plans for physical education, physical activities for the classroom (including video-led routines and afternoon activity breaks), and whole-school events and activities. The program is designed to be easy to use, engaging, and fun for teachers and students. More complete details are included in part I of this book.

**Fitness for Life: Elementary School** is the result of a team effort. Scott Wikgren, director of the Health, Physical Education, Recreation, and Dance division of Human Kinetics, was the driving force behind this project. He was responsible for bringing the successful and award-winning **Fitness for Life: High School** program to Human Kinetics and also was the driving force behind the award-winning **Fitness for Life: Middle School** program. With Scott's assistance, an author team and a team of expert consultants were assembled. Together, Scott and I chose Guy Le Masurier, Dolly Lambdin, and Meg Greiner as coauthors for the project. Ellen Abbadessa and Jeff Walkuski were chosen as consulting authors. Guy contributes youthful enthusiasm, an excellent ability to put words on paper in a meaningful way, and a practical understanding of the needs of school-age youth. Dolly, former President of the National Association for Sport and Physical Education (NASPE) and recipient of the

University of Texas' Massey Award for Excellence in Teacher Education, also brings years of practical experience working with both students and teachers, an understanding of pedagogical principles and curriculum planning, and sound leadership. Meg has been honored as a NASPE Elementary Physical Educator of the Year, Disney Outstanding Specialist Teacher, and a *USA Today* All-Star Teacher. She has years of practical experience and is known for her innovative methods of promoting physical activity for all children. Ellen, an elementary physical education teacher and supervisor, helped with all aspects of the program but particularly with the teacher resources. Jeff, known for his years as a professor of physical education pedagogy, also contributed to all aspects of the program but primarily contributed to the afternoon activities in the classroom guides and related teacher information in each classroom lesson.

Other consultants who contributed to the project are listed on the acknowledgments page (p. ix). The consultants provided field testing, critiques of activities and book content, and suggestions for revisions and improvement. Special thanks go out to Linda Coyle, the social studies, physical education, and health specialist for the Paradise Valley, Arizona, schools. We also thank her excellent physical education advisory committee members for their input at all stages of program development and for their help in field testing the program. Many of the **Fitness for Life** instructors who participate in a program jointly sponsored by Physical Best and Human Kinetics also provided input.

Finally, I (and my coauthors) cannot say enough about the excellent work done by our editors, Ray Vallese and Derek Campbell, and our video and audio production partners, Doug Fink, Chris Johns, and Roger Francisco. In many ways Ray was really a coauthor of the program; not only did he do excellent development work and project coordination, but he also contributed many ideas and excellent content. Derek contributed in many similar ways. Both editors worked long hours and were diligent far beyond the call of duty. Doug and Chris were the creative minds behind the video productions and deserve Oscars for their work. Roger is the real pro who provided us with the music and other audio resources necessary for making the project a success. We cannot thank these people enough for their hard work and attention to detail. We would also like to thank all of the other people at Human Kinetics who contributed to this team effort.

Charles B. "Chuck" Corbin

# ACKNOWLEDGMENTS

Many people played a role in the development of **Fitness for Life: Elementary School**. The following list credits the people who made this program possible. As noted in the preface, many others at Human Kinetics also contributed, and we acknowledge them all.

*Video (Human Kinetics)*
- Doug Fink, producer/director
- Roger Francisco, audio director
- Gregg Henness, camera operator/production assistant/teleprompter operator/Avid editor/DVD programmer
- Bill Yauch, camera operator
- Dan Walker, location audio
- Mark Herman, Avid editor/DVD programmer
- Chris Clark, Avid editor
- Sean Roosevelt, computer graphics art designer
- Stuart Cartwright, computer graphics art designer
- Amy Rose, production coordinator
- Chris Johns, scripts

*Video Production (Camera Originals, Oak Brook, Illinois)*
- Caren Cosby, producer/assistant director
- David Pierro, director of photography
- Dave Cosby, camera operator
- Tom McCosky, camera operator
- Ian Vacek, camera assistant
- Mark Markley, lighting
- Peter Horowitz, grip
- E.J. Huntemann, grip
- Dave Jack, audio technician
- Jackie Florczak, makeup/wardrobe
- Sarah Murphy, production coordinator
- Lauryn Kardatzke, production assistant
- Casey Lock, production assistant
- Kim Williams, O'Connor Casting

*Video Hosts (K-2)*
- David Goodloe
- Britni Tozzi

*Video Hosts (3-6)*
- Akula Lyman
- Laura Ball

*Video Messages (authors)*
- Chuck Corbin
- Guy Le Masurier
- Dolly Lambdin
- Meg Greiner
- Ellen Abbadessa (contributor)
- Jodi Le Masurier (contributor)

*Audio/Music (Human Kinetics)*
- Roger Francisco

*Music Lyrics*
- Chuck Corbin

*Lyrics Advisors*
- Cathie Corbin
- Dave Corbin
- Kris Youngkin
- Joan Milligan
- Dolly Lambdin

*All About Dance Studio*
- Jessica Goldman

*Dance Consultants*
- Josie Metal-Corbin
- Cathie Corbin
- Katie Corbin

- Julia Corbin
- Molly Corbin
- Suzi Corbin
- Joan Milligan

### Performers (K-2)

- Christopher Chu
- Rohan Jain
- Carlton Jenkins
- Alex Rich
- Hayden Whitley
- Vincent Wilkinson
- Princess Jenkins
- Olivia Klein
- Brooke Kolker
- Claire Seymour
- Mollie Smithson
- Emma Weiss
- Chloe Zoller

### Performers (3-6)

- Krystal Anderson
- Nair Banks
- Allie Bensinger
- Lauren Borg
- Caroline Chu
- Courtney Cosby
- Emily Schwartz
- Ashlyn Wiebe
- Aram Wilkinson
- Benjie Barclay
- Travis Little
- Kyle Birnbaum
- Nick Lucero
- Robert Banks

### Performers (Guide for Wellness Coordinators DVD)

- Mollee Carter
- Ana Martinez
- Jose Quiroz

- Heaven Reed
- Rufina Reutov
- Rolando Sifuentez

### Teacher Consultants

Paradise Valley, Arizona

- Linda Coyle, social studies, physical education & health, curriculum specialist
- Jay Thomas, Pinnacle High School
- Tonya Schwailler, Horizon High School
- Tammy Butler, Mountain Trail Middle School
- Craig Vogenson, Explorer Middle School
- Michael Wooldridge, Village Vista Elementary School
- Michele Popa, Desert Springs Elementary School
- Becki Griffen, Copper Canyon Elementary School
- George Mang, Pinnacle Peak Elementary School
- Susie Etchenbarren, PVUSD Adaptive Physical Education

Austin, Texas

- Laura Mikulencak, Pillow Elementary School
- Courtney Perry, Barton Hills Elementary School
- Tammy Arredondo, Graham Elementary School

Phoenix, Arizona

- Suzi Corbin

### Contributing Authors

- Ellen Abbadessa
- Jeff Walkuski

### Physical Best Authors

- Laura Borsdorf
- Lois Boeyink
- NASPE in association with AAHPERD

## Dance Credits

- Harvest Time: movements adapted, with permission, from a video of a traditional African harvest dance (Djole) by Charles Ahovissi.

- Tinikling: movements adapted from Corbin, C.B. (1969), *Becoming physically educated in the elementary school,* Philadelphia: Lea & Febiger, used by permission of author and copyright owner, pages 323-329.

- Jumpnastics: movements adapted from Corbin, C.B. & Corbin, D.E. (1972), *Inexpensive equipment for games, play and physical activity,* Dubuque, IA: Brown, used by permission of authors and copyright owners, pages 49-50.

- Stomp and Balance: adapted from the Danish dance Seven Jumps as described by Corbin, C.B. (1969), *Becoming physically educated in the elementary school,* Philadelphia: Lea & Febiger, used by permission of author and copyright owner, pages 308-309, credit to RCA records, 1958 for original permission (now out of print).

- Hip Hop 5: adapted from a routine created by Mychal Taylor, Cecily Taylor, and Josie Metal-Corbin, used by permission.

- Keep on Clapping: adapted from a routine created by Mychal Taylor, Cecily Taylor, and Josie Metal-Corbin, used by permission.

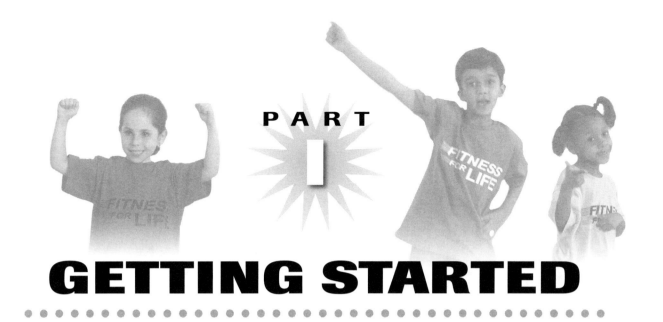

# PART

# 1

# GETTING STARTED

**P**art I of this guide provides a general introduction to the **Fitness for Life: Elementary School** program, a more detailed section on using the classroom lesson plans, and an executive summary.

- **Program Introduction** (page 3): This section introduces the **FFL: Elementary** program, discussing its rationale, organization, components, responsibilities, educational foundations, and overall philosophy.

- **Using the Lesson Plans** (page 13): This section outlines the responsibilities of the classroom teacher in providing morning and afternoon activity breaks, describes the lesson plan format, provides explanations of the elements in classroom lesson plans, and offers tips for successful delivery of the lessons.

- **Executive Summary** (page 19): This summary distills the program's rationale and main components into a single page.

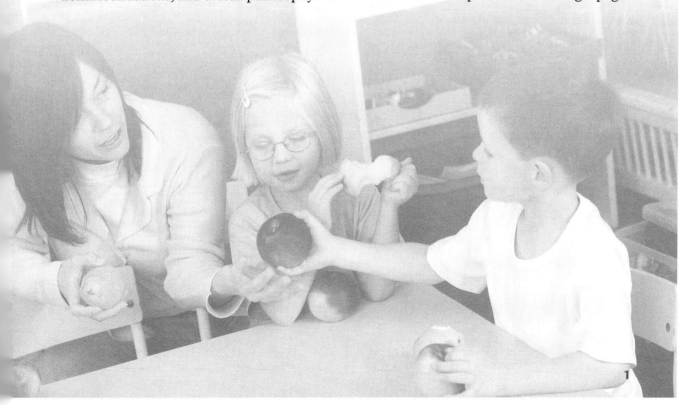

# PROGRAM INTRODUCTION

## Fitness for Life Elementary School

**F**itness for Life: Elementary School (FFL: Elementary) is a unique program that focuses on schoolwide wellness. It provides curriculum materials for the classroom and physical education classes, as well as schoolwide activities and take-home information that promote healthy lifestyles in the school and the community. The healthy lifestyles components feature sound nutrition and regular physical activity. The program is designed specifically for elementary school students and involves the entire school, including teachers, administrators, and staff.

## Program Rationale

Every school that receives federal school lunch program money must develop and carry out a school wellness policy. **FFL: Elementary** helps schools carry out a wellness plan. It supplements other school programs, such as physical education, health curricula, and school cafeteria programs. It provides a focal point for healthy lifestyle promotion on a schoolwide basis. Some important outcomes of **FFL: Elementary** include the following:

- **Helping children meet national physical activity guidelines**. National physical activity guidelines call for 60 minutes of physical activity each day for every child. Many youth do not get the recommended amount of activity (United States Department of Health and Human Services [USDHHS], 2008). **FFL: Elementary** helps students meet the guidelines and is especially important to children whose daily activity outside of school is low.

- **Helping children avoid becoming overweight or obese**. Childhood obesity has tripled since the 1980s. Today, more

Some of the information provided in this section is similar to information provided in the introduction to the *Physical Education Lesson Plans* and the *Guide for Wellness Coordinators*. This overlap is intentional. Not all teachers will read the same books, and it is important for everyone to get similar information. The *Guide for Wellness Coordinators* includes more detail about the **Fitness for Life: Elementary School** program and its educational foundations. Wellness coordinators may want to lend their guide to classroom teachers, physical education teachers, and others who want more information about the program.

than 15 percent of children are classified as obese, and an additional 15 percent or more are classified as overweight (Ogden et al., 2008). Regular physical activity and sound nutrition can contribute significantly to solving the problem.

- **Helping children avoid long periods of inactivity**. National guidelines indicate that children should not be inactive for long periods of time. We often condemn television watching and excessive use of computer games by children because they promote inactivity, yet schools often do the same thing—keep children inactive for long periods of time. Providing activity breaks and teaching children about physical activity and nutrition are good educational policies.
- **Helping children eat well**. Reinforcing sound nutrition in **FFL: Elementary**

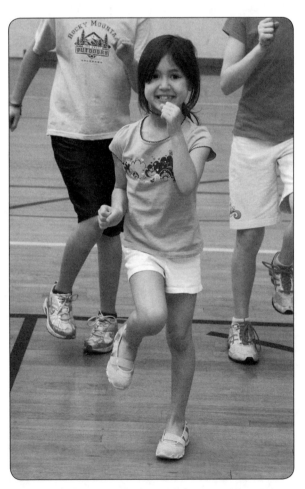

National physical activity guidelines call for 60 minutes of physical activity every day for every child.

programs can help children improve nutrition habits, help prevent obesity, and improve general health.

- **Enhancing academic achievement**. Recent evidence clearly shows that time taken during the school day to involve children in physical activity does not decrease academic learning. In fact, there is ample evidence that physical activity breaks during the day enhance academic learning (Hillman et al., 2009a; Hillman et al., 2009b; Le Masurier & Corbin, 2006; Ratey, 2008; Smith & Lounsbery, 2009).
- **Stimulating cognitive function.** Benefits of regular physical activity include improved blood flow and vascular supply to the brain and increased production of brain-derived neurotrophic factor (BDNF) that supports neural connections (Ratey, 2008).
- **Helping your school fulfill its wellness plan**. All schools receiving federal funding for school meal programs must have a school wellness policy and comply with it (Le Masurier & Corbin, 2006). Taking the time to include **FFL: Elementary** in your program will help you and your school meet the school wellness policy requirement.

## Program Organization

**Fitness for Life: Elementary School** is constructed to focus attention on physical activity and nutrition during four weeks of the school year. One week in every nine weeks of school is designated as Wellness Week. During each Wellness Week, the entire school focuses on wellness, emphasizing sound nutrition and regular physical activity. The exact dates of each Wellness Week are determined by the school staff. A wellness coordinator will be chosen to help coordinate the week's activities. In many cases, the physical education teacher will serve as wellness coordinator; however, the coordinator could be a classroom teacher, a nurse, a school staff member, or even a parent.

You may find the **FFL: Elementary** format so engaging and helpful that you want to include the activities every week, which would be great.

But the basic program involves classroom activities during one week of every nine weeks of school.

Each Wellness Week has two themes, one for physical activity and one for nutrition. Daily wellness messages are emphasized during Wellness Week. Table 1.1 illustrates the themes and messages for each Wellness Week. Special schoolwide nutrition activities are planned every Wednesday (Eat Well Wednesday), and schoolwide physical activities are planned every Friday (Get Fit Friday). You and your students will participate in these activities, which are organized by the wellness coordinator.

**Table 1.1 Messages for Each Wellness Week**

| Wellness Week | Activity theme | Nutrition theme | Daily messages for K-2 | Daily messages for 3-5 | Daily messages for 6 |
|---|---|---|---|---|---|
| Week 1 (held in fall, or during the first 9 weeks of the school year) | Moderate physical activity | Fruits and vegetables | 1: Be active every day. 2: Keep on trying. 3: Fitness foods 4: Play safely. 5: I can, you can, we all can. | 1: 60 minutes every day 2: The more you practice, the better you get. 3: Eat 5 a day. 4: Start with safety. 5: Fun for me, fun for you, fun for all. | 1: There are lots of fun physical activities. 2: Practice builds skills. 3: You are what you eat. 4: Safety is key for staying healthy. 5: I can! |
| Week 2 (held in fall/winter, or during the second 9 weeks of the school year) | Vigorous physical activity (vigorous aerobics, sports, and recreation) | Grains and high-calorie foods | 1: Get your body moving! 2: Get better with practice. 3: Foods with fats 4: Exercise your heart. 5: Never, ever give up! | 1: Play for a good day. 2: Build skills, have more fun. 3: Avoid empty calories. 4: Aerobic activity every day 5: Show respect. | 1: Active all day 2: Start with the basics. 3: High-calorie foods 4: Heartbeats for health 5: Self-respect |
| Week 3 (held in winter/spring, or during the third 9 weeks of the school year) | Muscle fitness and flexibility exercises | Protein | 1: Get your muscles ready. 2: Move your body. 3: Food for strong bones and muscles 4: You have only one body; make it fit! 5: If it is to be, it's up to me. | 1: Take care of your muscles. 2: Practice for fitness. 3: Protein power 4: Be specific; look terrific. 5: Don't be a character—have character. | 1: There is no "I" in "team". 2: Feedback to improve 3: Protein is important. 4: You get what you train for. 5: Rules rule! |
| Week 4 (held in spring, or during the fourth 9 weeks of the school year) | Integration (energy balance) | Energy balance | 1: Get off your seat and move your feet. 2: Play lots, learn lots. 3: Healthy food helps us move. 4: Be water wise. 5: Plan to get better. | 1: Brain and body exercise 2: Combine skills just for the fun of it. 3: Balance energy in (food) with energy out (exercise). 4: Water, water, before I get hotter! 5: Personal fitness starts with you. | 1: Build a healthy body; build a healthy mind. 2: One step at a time 3: Balance calories. 4: Hit the water. 5: SMART goals |

This table presents the overall nutrition theme for each Wellness Week; each grade range has a more specific variation of that theme. For example, the K-2 nutrition theme for Wellness Week 1 is "Fruits and vegetables (fitness foods)."

# WHAT IS WELLNESS?

The **Fitness for Life: Elementary School** program focuses on wellness for school children. It includes Wellness Week activities that can be used to implement wellness policy as mandated by federal law. To implement an effective wellness program, it is helpful to have a clear understanding of the meaning of the word *wellness*. Many years ago, the World Health Organization defined health as being more than absence of disease (WHO, 1947). It was agreed that wellness, not just sickness, should be included in a definition of good health. The characteristics of wellness include the following:

* Wellness is part of good health.
* Wellness is a state of being exemplified by quality of life and a sense of well-being. Examples of quality of life and a sense of well-being from the health goals for our nation include the ability to perform activities of daily life without restriction, happiness, satisfaction with our lives, self-esteem, and a positive outlook on life.
* Wellness is considered the positive component of good health (more than freedom from illness).
* Health and its positive component (wellness) are integrated; each interacts with the other, and if one is influenced, both are influenced.
* Both health and wellness are multidimensional. The most commonly described dimensions are physical, social, intellectual, emotional (mental), and spiritual.

Two healthy lifestyles prominent in **FFL: Elementary** are regular physical activity and sound nutrition. These two lifestyles have been shown to have a positive impact on wellness and to reduce the risk of chronic diseases. Especially important is the fact that regular physical activity and sound nutrition are factors in life over which people have control. For this reason, these two behaviors are considered to be high-priority lifestyles. They can be changed with the help of educators and sound educational programs such as **FFL: Elementary**. Those who adopt healthy lifestyles will have improved health and wellness. Wellness programs typically include an emphasis on physical activity and nutrition because of their known benefits to personal wellness.

Adapted from Corbin, C.B., & Pangrazi, R.P. 2001. Toward a uniform definition of wellness: A commentary. *President's Council on Physical Fitness and Sports Research Digest, 3*(15), 1-8. Available at www.fitness.gov/publications/digests/pcpfs_research_digs.html.

## Program Components

The components of Wellness Week include the following:

* **Classroom activity breaks using video routines** created especially for **FFL: Elementary**. The lesson plans for using these routines are provided in the classroom guide for each grade, and the routines are included on the DVD bound into each guide.

* **Classroom activity breaks using additional activities** that reinforce academic concepts in subjects such as math, science, and language arts. Plans for these breaks are included in the classroom guide for each grade.

- **Physical education lesson plans,** including one warm-up lesson for use the week before each Wellness Week and three lesson plans for use during each Wellness Week. These lesson plans are provided in the book *Physical Education Lesson Plans.*

- **Conceptual learning discussions** related to wellness (focusing on nutrition and physical activity) using messages on the DVD video routines. These are done in the classroom and in physical education class.

- **Signs** for the classroom, the gym, the cafeteria, and school bulletin boards promoting sound nutrition and regular physical activity. These are provided among the resource materials for each book.

- **Chants** to reinforce the major messages of each lesson.

- **Eat Well Wednesdays** that feature schoolwide nutrition activities (involving the cafeteria). The general nutrition themes for each Wellness Week are shown in table 1.1. The wellness coordinator works with the cafeteria staff to conduct the special nutrition activities.

- **Get Fit Fridays** that feature schoolwide physical activities called TEAM Time; TEAM stands for "Together Everyone Achieves More." The TEAM Time activities are organized by the wellness coordinator with the help of all school staff.

- **Other schoolwide events** (celebration activities) promoting sound nutrition and regular physical activity. These are coordinated by the wellness coordinator with the help of all school staff.

- **Newsletters** for distribution to families during Wellness Week. It is recommended that these be printed by the wellness coordinator and administrative staff and distributed to teachers for distribution to parents. However, they can also be printed at the classroom level or sent to parents by e-mail. Newsletters are provided among the resource materials for each book and can be customized to suit local needs.

- **Worksheets** for use in promoting sound nutrition and physical activity. Worksheets are used in the classroom and in physical education, and they are provided among the resource materials for each book.

- **FFL: Elementary Web site**. A Web site dedicated to **FFL: Elementary** is available at www.fitnessforlife.org. This site provides information for teachers, students, and parents.

# Program Responsibilities

Responsibilities for different members of the school staff are listed below. Duties for the classroom teacher are listed first.

### *Classroom Teacher*

- Conducts activity breaks in the classroom using video routines on the DVD included with this guide.

- Conducts discussions about wellness messages included on the videos.

- Conducts integrated activities in math, science, and other academic content areas as activity breaks (as outlined in the lesson plans in this guide).

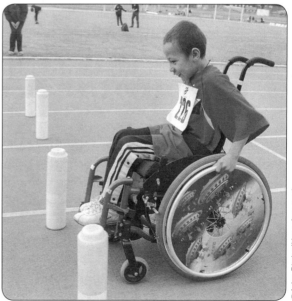

©John Birdsall/age fotostock

The **Fitness for Life: Elementary School** program provides activity for all children.

- Conducts the classroom discussion for Eat Well Wednesday.
- Posts the Wellness Week signs (on the DVD) in the classroom.
- Sends home the Wellness Week newsletter (provided by the wellness coordinator or printed from the DVD).
- Uses classroom worksheets (on the DVD) as appropriate.
- Assists with events planned by the wellness coordinator (e.g., Eat Well Wednesday, Get Fit Friday, celebration activities).

### School Principal

- Appoints or aids in selection of the wellness coordinator.
- Provides enthusiastic support for the **FFL: Elementary** program.
- Participates in schoolwide Wellness Week activities.

### Wellness Coordinator

- Conducts faculty–staff meeting to explain Wellness Week (uses PowerPoint® file on the *Guide for Wellness Coordinators* DVD).
- Coordinates Wellness Week activities.
- Oversees schoolwide events such as Eat Well Wednesday and Get Fit Friday activities.

- Distributes materials to teachers and staff (e.g., Wellness Week newsletters, plans for Wellness Week schoolwide events).
- Provides in-service as necessary.

### Physical Education Teacher

- Teaches the warm-up lesson the week before each Wellness Week. This includes teaching the video routine to be performed in the classroom during Wellness Week.
- Teaches lessons during Wellness Week.
- Posts Wellness Week signs in the gym or multipurpose room.
- Assists with schoolwide events planned by the wellness coordinator (e.g., Eat Well Wednesday, Get Fit Friday, celebration activities).
- May serve as the wellness coordinator—if so, performs duties listed above. The *Guide for Wellness Coordinators* provides more details.

### Art Teacher

- Works with the wellness coordinator and classroom teachers to promote wellness, physical activity, and nutrition during each Wellness Week.
- Has students create art related to wellness for posting on school walls. Consider a wellness art show.

# HOW WILL I FIND THE TIME TO DO ACTIVITIES IN MY CLASSROOM?

The authors of **Fitness for Life: Elementary School** are well aware of the time demands on teachers and the scarcity of time for meeting daily instructional goals. That is why it was decided to focus on the program for one week in every nine-week period. On each day during each Wellness Week, the classroom teacher will devote 5 to 15 minutes to the program for five consecutive days. *Taking 1 to 3 minutes from each hour of the school day (or 1 to 3 minutes from five different activities during the day) will give you the time.* Research shows that the time taken will not only improve student health and fitness but will also contribute to achievement in the classroom and to better test performance (Hillman et al., 2009a; Hillman et al., 2009b; Le Masurier & Corbin, 2006; Ratey, 2008; Smith & Lounsbery, 2009).

*Music Teacher*

- Works with classroom and physical education teachers to promote wellness during Wellness Week.
- Helps students learn songs from the classroom guide video routines (on the DVD) to be performed in the classroom.

*Librarian/Computer Teacher*

- Identifies books on wellness, nutrition, and physical activity and encourages students to read them during Wellness Week.
- Supports computer activities related to Wellness Week (e.g., MyPyramid Tracker, Activitygram).

*Nutrition Staff*

- Conducts schoolwide nutrition activities on Eat Well Wednesday.
- Posts Wellness Week nutrition signs in the school and cafeteria.

*Other Staff*

- Assist the wellness coordinator with schoolwide events.
- Assist in printing and posting Wellness Week signs.

*Parents*

- Help with schoolwide events.

- Encourage children to be active and eat well, especially during Wellness Week.

# Educational Foundations

**Fitness for Life: Elementary School** was created based on sound educational foundations. Some of the key information that was considered in building the program is summarized below. More comprehensive coverage of the educational foundations for **FFL: Elementary** is available in part III of the *Guide for Wellness Coordinators*. If you are interested in learning more about these foundations, borrow the guide from your wellness coordinator.

## Child Nutrition and WIC Reauthorization Act

In 2004, the United States Congress passed the Child Nutrition and Women, Infants and Children (WIC) Reauthorization Act (Public Law 108-265). As a result of the act, all states, school districts, and schools receiving funding for school lunch programs must have a policy (plan) designed to encourage total school wellness. Central to a sound wellness policy is the notion that the primary mission of schools is to promote optimal learning for all children, and this cannot be achieved if students are not fit, healthy, and well. **FFL: Elementary** helps

## EAT 5 TO 9 A DAY

To encourage consumption of a variety of fruits and vegetables, the **FFL: Elementary** program uses the simple "5 to 9 servings a day" message that is designed to help children meet national recommendations. For cooked vegetables, 1/2 cup equals one serving, and for leafy vegetables, 1 cup equals one serving. One medium apple, banana, or pear equals one fruit serving. The Centers for Disease Control and Prevention (CDC) uses the "Fruits & Veggies–More Matters" campaign to encourage more fruits and veggies in the diet. For more information, visit the following Web sites:

- ∗ www.fruitsandveggiesmatter.gov
- ∗ www.mypyramid.gov/pyramid/fruits_counts.html
- ∗ www.mypyramid.gov/pyramid/vegetables_counts.html

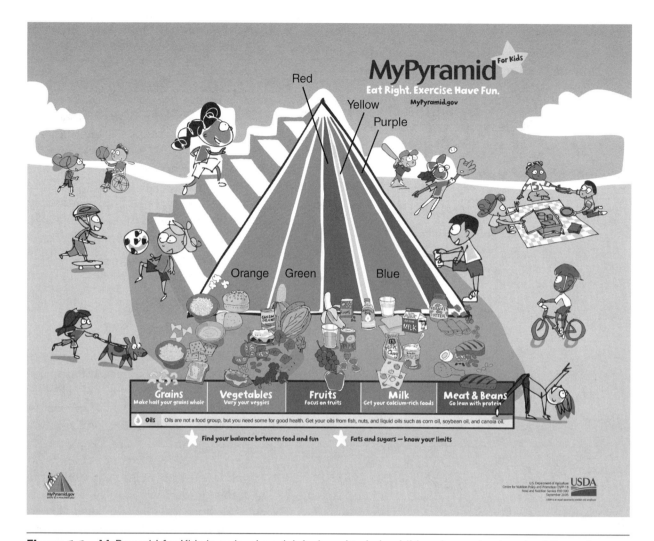

**Figure 1.1**   MyPyramid for Kids is a visual model designed to help children learn about each of the major food groups. MyPyramid is used extensively in the **FFL: Elementary** program. For more information go to www.mypyramid.gov.

Adapted from U.S. Department of Agriculture.

schools meet key guidelines of the legislation and can help your school meet wellness planning guidelines. Action for Healthy Kids is a national group dedicated to promoting school wellness and has many online tools to help implement school wellness plans. For more information, log on to www.actionforhealthykids.org.

## USDA National Nutrition Guidelines

Every five years a committee of the United States Department of Agriculture (USDA) revises the National Nutrition Guidelines. A recent revision resulted in the development of MyPyramid (see figure 1.1). The nutrition component of the **FFL:**

**Elementary** program relies heavily on information associated with MyPyramid for Kids. The steps on the side of MyPyramid for Kids represent the various forms of physical activity that are also depicted in the Physical Activity Pyramid for Kids (see figure 1.2). The USDA nutrition guidelines emphasize the importance of physical activity, together with sound nutrition, in promoting health and wellness.

## Physical Activity Pyramid for Kids

The Physical Activity Pyramid for Kids (see figure 1.2) illustrates the different types of physical activity that can be used to promote good

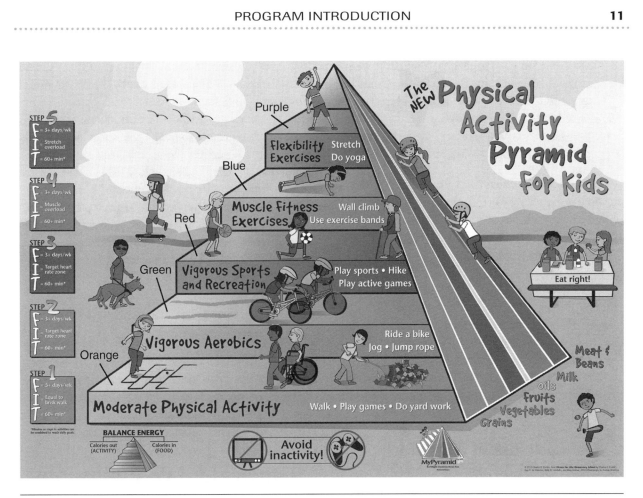

**Figure 1.2** The Physical Activity Pyramid for Kids is a visual model designed to help children learn about the five major physical activity types.

©2010 Charles B. Corbin

health, fitness, and wellness. The basic pyramid is used in all **Fitness for Life** programs, but there is a special version just for young children; the upper-level programs use the Physical Activity Pyramid for Teens. The Physical Activity Pyramid for Kids helps children better understand the benefits of the different types of activity. As noted earlier, each of the four Wellness Weeks focuses on a different type of physical activity from the pyramid.

The Physical Activity Pyramid for Kids has five colored steps that represent different types of activity.

- Moderate activity is represented by step 1 (orange). It includes activities equal to brisk walking, including active play for children. It is at the base of the pyramid because it is the most commonly performed activity and can be done regularly by all people.

- Step 2 (green) includes vigorous aerobics. Activities that are vigorous enough to elevate the heart rate in the heart rate target zone are considered to be vigorous aerobics. Jogging, biking at a relatively fast pace, and lap swimming are examples.

- Step 3 (red) includes vigorous sports and recreation such as tennis, soccer, and hiking. Only activities that elevate the heart rate sufficiently are considered to be vigorous in nature. Some sports and recreational activities such as bowling are classified as moderate (step 1).

- Step 4 (blue) includes exercises for muscle fitness. Climbing on a climbing structure, calisthenics such as push-ups or curl-ups, elastic band exercises, and stunts that require the use of arms and legs to move the body (e.g., crab walk) are examples of muscle fitness exercises.

- Step 5 (purple) includes flexibility exercises. Activities that require the muscles to stretch beyond their normal length are called flexibility exercises. Examples are gymnastics stunts, yoga, and stretching calisthenics (e.g., sit and reach).

National guidelines for children recommend activity from all steps of the pyramid. Inactivity or sedentary living is shown below the pyramid. Extended periods of inactivity (e.g., watching TV, playing inactive computer games) should be avoided.

The DVD in this guide includes a color version of the pyramid shown in figure 1.2. The pyramid is provided as one of the general signs for use during any Wellness Week (see page 17 for details about the general signs).

Part III of the *Guide for Wellness Coordinators* provides more details on the Physical Activity Pyramid for Kids.

## USDHHS National Physical Activity Guidelines for Children

In October of 2008, the USDHHS published national physical activity guidelines for children. These guidelines, as abstracted below, were used in developing the **FFL: Elementary** program. For more details, visit www.health.gov/paguidelines.

- Children should perform physical activity 60 minutes (or more) each day. Choose from either moderate (equal in intensity to brisk walking) or vigorous activity (activity that elevates heart rate).
- Children should perform vigorous activity at least 3 days per week.
- Children should perform stretching and muscle fitness activities that build muscles and bones at least 3 days per week.
- Activities should be age appropriate, enjoyable, and varied.

## NASPE Physical Education Curriculum Standards

The National Association for Sport and Physical Education (NASPE) has developed standards for the physical education curriculum. These standards have been used by 48 of the 50 states in developing state standards and physical education curricula and define the content needed to help individuals to have "the knowledge, skills and confidence to enjoy a lifetime of healthy physical activity" (NASPE, 2004). The lesson plans later in this book identify NASPE standards associated with each educational activity. A description of the six primary NASPE standards and the performance outcomes used to build the **FFL: Elementary** program are included in appendix B.

## Curriculum Standards for Other Academic Areas

Curriculum standards in other areas such as math were considered in developing **FFL: Elementary** lessons. A more detailed description of these standards is included in appendix B and at www.EducationWorld.com.

## Fitness for Life Philosophy

**Fitness for Life: Elementary School** is part of a comprehensive K-12 program. In addition to **FFL: Elementary**, there are **Fitness for Life** programs for middle school and high school (see www.fitnessforlife.org for details). All **Fitness for Life** programs are based on the **HELP** philosophy. The first letters in four key words form the **HELP** acronym.

- **H**ealth. The program is designed to help elementary school students learn about health-related physical fitness and the benefits of healthy lifestyles, including regular physical activity and sound nutrition.
- **E**veryone. The program is designed for everyone (all elementary school students), not just those with special physical talents.
- **L**ifetime. The activities included in all **Fitness for Life** programs were chosen to get kids active now as well as build habits that will last a lifetime.
- **P**ersonal. All lessons are designed to help each student learn personally appropriate physical activity and nutrition information.

# USING THE LESSON PLANS

Part II of this book, starting on page 21, presents lesson plans for each day of each Wellness Week. Each component of the lesson plans is described below, along with suggestions concerning how to use the plans.

## Introduction to Wellness Week

Each Wellness Week begins with a short introduction that summarizes the week's activities, themes, standards, resources (signs, worksheets, newsletters, and Web sites), and special days (Eat Well Wednesday and Get Fit Friday). This introduction also identifies the standards that are met by the activities. The NASPE physical education standards and sample performance indicators are listed by their abbreviations (e.g., 1A, 2B) in the introduction to each Wellness Week, and complete descriptions of these standards appear in appendix B.

By design, the lesson plans for each Wellness Week have some common components. Plans for each week are comprehensive so that you will not have to refer back to previous lessons to find information. Each set of lesson plans provides everything that you will need for each Wellness Week.

## Lesson Plan Template

Each lesson plan provided in **FFL: Elementary** follows the same general format. That format is described below. Some sections of the lesson plans include text in quotation marks, which is material that is meant to be spoken (or paraphrased) to students.

### Overview

The lesson plan overview provides the names of activities that can be used for five-minute morning and afternoon activity breaks and that day's message. The morning breaks are movement routines led by the video, and the afternoon breaks are simple activities designed to get students active as well as have them practice basic math or science concepts such as patterns, categorizing, matching, and sequencing.

### Objectives

Here, specific objectives for the lesson (based on the previously described standards) are listed.

### Resources

This part of the lesson plan provides a list of the resources (from the DVD that accompanies this guide) needed to conduct the lesson. In addition to video routines for use in classroom activity breaks, the DVD includes signs for posting in the classroom, worksheets for teaching wellness concepts, and newsletters that promote wellness, physical activity, and sound nutrition that can be printed and sent home to parents. See "Using the DVD" later in this section for more details.

## Morning Activity Break

This part of the lesson plan describes how to use the DVD to conduct a morning activity break in the classroom. Each week, the students perform a different activity routine. The same routine is repeated all five days of the week, but the routines provide new health and wellness messages every day. Each routine follows a simple pattern: The video hosts deliver an introductory message, students watch the routine and follow along, the hosts deliver a middle message, students perform the routine again, and finally the hosts deliver a concluding message.

After the routine, you will lead a discussion about the concepts introduced in the messages, using the background information and discussion questions provided. The lesson plan also offers suggestions for closure.

If your school has a physical education teacher, he or she may have taught the routine to students during the week before Wellness Week. If not, an instructional video is provided to help you teach the routine.

## Chants

Chanting is a great way to reinforce a message. For each chant, the lesson plan provides a teacher phrase and a student response phrase. The first time you try a chant, you'll need to tell students that when you say the teacher phrase, they should respond by saying the student response phrase. Practice it three or four times the first time you introduce each new chant. The chants are on the signs, so if you print and post the signs, you can use the chants whenever you want throughout the day.

## Afternoon Activity Break

The lesson plan contains ideas for a simple but active afternoon activity break that can be done in place in the classroom. These activities do not use the DVD. They provide practice in patterns, categorizing, matching, and sequencing.

## Additional Activities

At the end of each lesson is a reminder to look in appendix A for additional enriching activities that integrate drawing, writing, measuring, data collection, and graphing with physical activities. The enrichment activities can be used as

## FIVE DAYS A WEEK

Each Wellness Week includes five lesson plans, referred to as Day 1, Day 2, Day 3, Day 4, and Day 5. Typically, during each week, Day 1 will be Monday, Day 2 will be Tuesday, and so on. However, for simplicity, the lesson plans refer only to Day 1, Day 2, and so on. This approach will also help you keep the lessons in order if a day is missed. Remember, too, about the Wellness Week special days:

 * On Day 3 of each week (usually Wednesday), the lesson includes a section called Eat Well Wednesday. This section presents a mini-lesson

on nutrition and provides a reminder about the schoolwide nutrition activity (planned by the wellness coordinator) that takes place on Wednesday. If necessary, this information could be presented on a day other than Wednesday.

 * On Day 5 of each week (usually Friday), the lesson includes a section called Get Fit Friday. This section provides a reminder about the schoolwide physical activity (planned by the wellness coordinator) that takes place on Friday. If necessary, the activity could be presented on a day other than Friday.

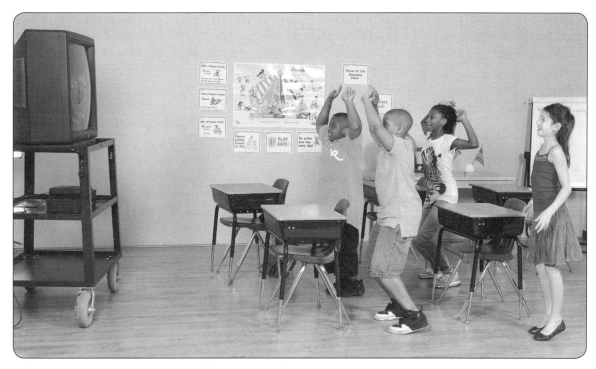

Physical activity breaks during the day help children avoid long periods of inactivity while learning valuable messages about nutrition and physical activity.

an alternative to the afternoon activity break or as an additional activity break during the day.

# Icons for Effective Teaching Practices

Throughout the lesson plans, you will encounter icons that signal opportunities to enhance your teaching of the lesson.

You can use these strategies for assessing student learning and student participation. You may want to come up with a system on your roll sheet for identifying student understanding and student behavior for assessment purposes.

**Teacher Tip**: This icon is accompanied by a suggestion that you may want to consider when delivering the lesson.

**Review**: Whenever you encounter this icon in the lesson plans, we have provided suggestions for reviewing key lesson concepts or concepts from a previous lesson. As you deliver the lessons, you may find that there are many more situations where reviewing key concepts or class protocols would enhance the lesson.

**Comprehension Check**: Whenever you encounter this icon in the lesson plans, we have provided suggestions for checking students' understanding of the class content, instructions, or demonstrations. You may find many more opportunities during the lessons where a check for student understanding would be helpful. In his textbook, *Teaching Children Physical Education, Third Edition,* George Graham (2008) outlines five approaches to checking for understanding:

- *Recognition check*: A quick way to check for student understanding is to ask students to raise their hands, give a thumbs up or down, or hold up a response card (e.g., A, B, C, or D) to indicate that the concept, instruction, or demonstration was understood.

- *Verbal check*: Ask students to tell you the concept or cue you are teaching.

- *Comprehension check*: Ask students to explain the concept. This shows a deeper understanding than a verbal check.

- *Performance check*: Ask the students to demonstrate the activity, skill, principle, and so on. If all students perform at once, this check allows you to see at a glance who understands the concept and who needs additional help.

• *Closure*: At the end of the lesson, you can use a short closure session to get an idea of how well students have learned lesson concepts. During the one- to two-minute closure session, bring students together to review key points, get student comments, or prepare for assignments or the next class.

(icon) **Observation:** This icon identifies a point in the lesson plans where observation of student behavior may be appropriate. By looking around the room, you can easily determine if students are on task, working together, performing movements correctly, and following instructions. You will often see this icon when students are asked to work cooperatively in group settings. We believe it is important to celebrate respectful communication (listening and talking) and inclusion of different points of view.

(icon) **Interdisciplinary:** This icon identifies a point in the lesson where other academic subjects could be integrated with the activity.

# Using the DVD

The DVD bound into the back of this guide includes the daily video routines, the instructional videos that teach the movements for the routines, and the resources for use with the lesson plans. The last page of this guide provides the technical details for using the DVD. This section explains how to use the videos and resources.

Like the lesson plans, the resources are designed to meet the standards associated with the separate grade ranges. Thus, grades K-2 share the same resources, grades 3-5 share the same resources, and grade 6 has its own resources.

**The contents of the DVD, including all videos and resources, are intended for use only by instructors and agencies that have purchased this classroom guide. The reproduction of the contents of the DVD is otherwise forbidden according to the terms stated on the copyright page of this guide.**

## Videos

When you insert the DVD in a DVD player, the TV screen will display a menu of video routines to use during the morning activity breaks (as described under "Morning Activity Break" on page 14). There are six closed-captioned videos per week: one instructional video and five daily routines that reinforce different wellness messages throughout the week. The lesson plans will direct you to play the correct video each day.

Each Wellness Week, each grade will perform a different routine. The routines are designed to reinforce the weekly physical activity theme. Table 1.2 shows the routines for all grades.

## Table 1.2  Routines by Grade Level

| Grade | Week 1<br>Theme: Moderate<br>physical activity | Week 2<br>Theme: Vigorous<br>physical activity | Week 3<br>Theme: Muscle fitness<br>and flexibility exercises | Week 4<br>Theme: Integration<br>(energy balance) |
|---|---|---|---|---|
| K | Exercise on the Farm | Frank and Franny Fitness | We Get Fit | Shake It |
| 1 | Some More | I Can | CYIM Fit | Stomp and Balance |
| 2 | Get Fit | La Raspa | Wave It | It's the One |
| 3 | It's Our Plan | Go Aerobics Go | Tic Tac Toe 3 | Jumpnastics |
| 4 | Robot | Latin Aerobics | Tic Tac Toe 4 | Keep on Clapping |
| 5 | Hip Hop 5 | Tinikling | Tic Tac Toe 5 | Fit Funk |
| 6 | Hip Hop 6 | Salsaerobics | Tic Tac Toe 6 | Harvest Time |

## Resources

When you access the DVD through your computer's DVD-ROM drive, you will see a folder called Resources. Inside it are five folders of resources: General, Wellness Week 1, Wellness Week 2, Wellness Week 3, and Wellness Week 4.

### General

This folder contains general **Fitness for Life: Elementary School** signs related to physical activity and nutrition. The messages and concepts in these signs are discussed in classrooms and in physical education classes and are included in video routine messages. Posting the general signs on bulletin boards and in hallways will help reinforce what students are learning in program activities. Review the general signs and choose several to post during each Wellness Week. The folder contains 13 files:

Blank horizontal

Blank vertical

Executive Summary

G1: Fitness for Life: Elementary School

G2: Wellness Week

G3: Physical Activity Pyramid for Kids

G4: MyPyramid for Kids

G5: Eat Well Wednesday

G6: TEAM Time: Together Everyone Achieves More

G7: Get Fit Friday

G8: Healthy mind, healthy body, healthy heart . . . let's start!

G9: ABCs of Physical Activity (signs for each letter of the alphabet, including two signs for the letter M)

G10: ABCs of Nutrition (signs for each letter of the alphabet)

When using the general signs, you can print all the signs at once and save them to reuse during future Wellness Weeks. You can also put specific classes in charge of managing special bulletin boards where the signs are posted each week.

The general signs are PDF files and can be printed but not edited. For this reason, we have provided two blank signs that feature the **Fitness for Life: Elementary School** design but that have no message content. You can print these blank signs and customize them as desired, either by hand or by feeding the signs back through your printer.

Throughout this guide, references to general signs are accompanied by the following icon to remind you of where to find the signs on the DVD:

 **General**

### Wellness Week Resources

The DVD includes one folder of resources for each Wellness Week. Each of these folders contains three subfolders:

• The newsletter to be used during that week

• Signs to be used during that week

• Worksheets to be used during that week

In the Signs folder, the signs for the week are grouped into one PDF file to make it easy for you to print them all at once. For example, the file called "K-2 signs week 1" contains all the classroom signs needed for Wellness Week 1.

Similarly, in the Worksheets folder, the worksheets for the week are grouped into one PDF file. For grades 3, 4, 5, and 6, the worksheets

## PRINTING SIGNS

Because the signs in these folders are intended to be engaging, they are presented in color, but they will print normally to black-and-white printers as well. If you have a color printer but wish to conserve your color ink, you can print the signs in grayscale. (Every printer is different, so for details on how to do this, check your printer's instruction manual, or click the Help or Properties button in your Print window.)

folder contains worksheets that teach and reinforce wellness concepts. For grades K-2, the worksheets are for students to color and decorate. Included are black-and-white versions of MyPyramid for Kids, the Physical Activity Pyramid for Kids, and all of the classroom signs without graphics.

Finally, the Newsletter folder contains the newsletter for use during the week. Each newsletter is a document, not a PDF file, so that you can customize it using your favorite word processing software. Ideally, your school's wellness coordinator will customize the newsletter and distribute copies to teachers to send home with students. Alternatively, the newsletter can be customized by a classroom teacher or physical education teacher, and it can be sent to families by e-mail.

Throughout this guide, references to Wellness Week resources are accompanied by the following icons to remind you of where to find the resources on the DVD:

 **Wellness Week 1 → Signs**

 **Wellness Week 1 → Worksheets**

 **Wellness Week 1 → Newsletter**

## Tips for Using the Lesson Plans

The lesson plans have been designed to be easy to use. They are brief so that you can refer to them as you are teaching. The morning activity breaks will use videos you can play for the children to follow. The children may have learned the week's video routine in physical education class the week before. If not, you can substitute the instructional version for the Day 1 video on Monday and let them learn it as they go.

In any teaching it is important to have good protocols, and **Fitness for Life: Elementary School** is no exception. Talk to the children before starting an activity. Let them know where you want them to stand and what they should do when they finish the routine. Explain that they should practice deep breathing at the end of each activity and pay attention to the feelings in their healthy body—not collapse on the floor! Talk to

them about how important it is to control their movements and teach them how to move safely so they won't hit anyone else. Then have them stand and move a little while you provide lots of praise for safe movements. As you know, a little preparation makes everything go more smoothly.

Below is a list of simple steps to ensure a great experience from the first time onward.

- Prior to conducting each lesson, first review the standards for the week, the lesson overview, and the lesson objectives.
- Gather the required materials (usually just the DVD player and monitor) and print teacher resources that will be used that day (e.g., signs, newsletters, and worksheets).
- Morning Activity Break: Prior to the lesson, view the DVD video routine for the day. There is a separate video for each of the five days of the Wellness Week. Each video contains different daily messages but contains the same video routine for all five days. Read over the background information, discussion questions, and closure statements associated with this activity.
- Afternoon Activity Break: Read the directions for the afternoon activity break as well as the directions for the other enriching activities.

The K-6 lesson plans are designed to allow for grade level progression. In K-2, children will be learning some basic concepts, participating in physical activity, and following the video and teacher directions. The lesson plans are structured so that as children progress from grades 3 to 5, they will take over some of the leader positions. By the fifth or sixth grade, the students should be essentially leading the program by posting the signs, creating their own chants and signs, and leading the activity breaks.

> The Executive Summary on the next page provides an overview of the **Fitness for Life: Elementary School** program. A PDF file of the summary is available on the DVD. It can be printed and distributed to school staff, parents, and others who are interested in the program.

# EXECUTIVE SUMMARY

## What Is Fitness for Life: Elementary School?

Fitness for Life: Elementary School (**FFL: Elementary**) is a program designed to promote wellness, physical activity, sound nutrition, and healthy lifestyles throughout the entire school.

## Why Should I Do the Program?

Some of the principal benefits of **FFL: Elementary** are as follows:

* Helps your students meet national physical activity guidelines.
* Helps your school implement a wellness policy as required by law.
* Helps prevent childhood obesity by teaching about expending calories and limiting caloric intake.
* Helps build youth fitness.
* Helps children eat a healthy diet and meet national nutrition goals.
* Promotes academic achievement.
* Stimulates activity that increases blood flow to the brain.

## What Are the Basic Components of the Program?

**FFL: Elementary** is a schoolwide wellness program that requires participation by all school employees and students. Once every nine weeks, the entire school conducts a Wellness Week (four each year). Major activities of each Wellness Week include the following:

* **Classroom activity breaks** that use teacher-friendly DVD videos and lesson plans
* **Physical education activities** that use provided lesson plans

* **Schoolwide special events** with plans for Eat Well Wednesday (a day of nutrition activities), Get Fit Friday (a day of TEAM Time physical activities), and celebration activities
* **School signs** promoting wellness to be posted throughout the school
* **Educational video messages** that teach children about wellness, sound nutrition, and physical activity
* **Worksheets** to reinforce learning about sound nutrition and physical activity
* **Newsletters** to help families get involved in Wellness Week
* A **Web site** to help students and families learn more about important wellness concepts

## How Do I Find Time for the Program?

Time is at a premium in elementary school, and there are many educational goals to be met. So how can you find the time for **FFL: Elementary**? The program is conducted during four weeks each year so that a concentrated effort can be placed on wellness during these specific weeks. The classroom activity breaks can be done in 5 to 6 minutes. The total time for **FFL: Elementary** is 10 to 15 minutes per day. Research shows that time in physical activity can promote learning in the classroom, so the time is well spent. The breaks also promote fitness, health, and wellness. Taking 2 to 3 minutes from each hour of the school day will provide the time to conduct classroom activity breaks. The physical education lessons can be conducted in regular physical education classes and can be integrated with the regular physical education program.

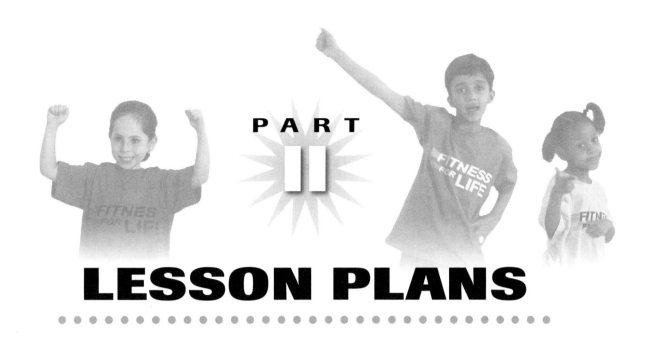

# PART II

# LESSON PLANS

$P$art II contains the **Fitness for Life: Elementary School** lesson plans for second grade, organized by Wellness Week. Before you use the lesson plans, be sure to read part I (especially "Using the Lesson Plans," starting on page 13) and familiarize yourself with the classroom videos and resources on the DVD that accompanies this guide.

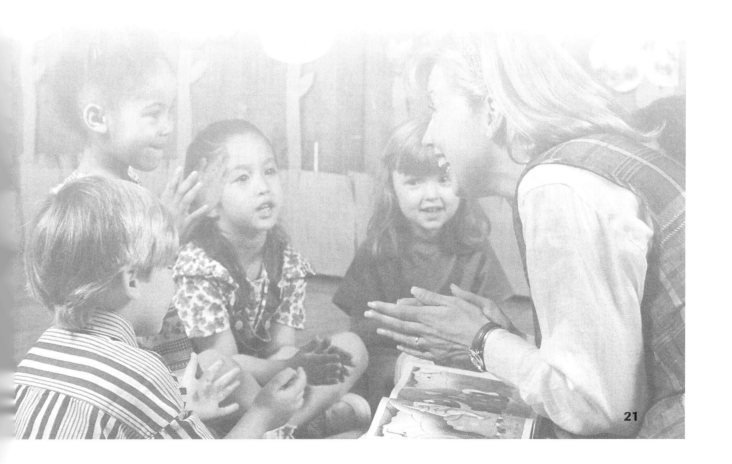

# WELLNESS WEEK 1

## Fitness for Life Elementary School

## Week 1 Overview

Table 2.1 is a summary chart of the Wellness Week 1 activities for the second grade classroom. Pages 27 through 50 provide the daily lesson plans for each day of week 1.

- Week 1 physical activity theme: Moderate physical activity
- Week 1 nutrition theme: Fruits and vegetables (fitness foods)

## Week 1 NASPE Standards

Week 1 activities meet the National Association for Sport and Physical Education (NASPE) standards listed here. For full standards and specific performance indicators (e.g., 1A through 6G), see appendix B.

- Standard 1: Motor skills and movement patterns, 1A, 1B, 1C, 1E, 1F
- Standard 2: Movement concepts and principles, 2C, 2D

**Table 2.1  Summary of Wellness Week 1 Activities**

| Activity | Day 1 Monday | Day 2 Tuesday | Day 3 Wednesday | Day 4 Thursday | Day 5 Friday |
|---|---|---|---|---|---|
| Morning Activity Break | Video routine performed every day of the week: Get Fit | | | | |
| Daily Message | Be active every day. | Keep on trying. | Fitness foods | Play safely. | I can, you can, we all can. |
| Afternoon Activity Break | Head, Shoulders, Knees, and Toes | Pattern Practice | Simon Says | Follow the Leader | Alphabet Lineup |
| Eat Well Wednesday Classroom Discussion | — | — | Track Your Fruits and Veggies | — | — |
| Schoolwide Events | — | — | Eat Well Wednesday: A to Z Fruit and Veggie Bar in the Cafeteria | — | Get Fit Friday: TEAM Time 1: School Walk |

23

- Standard 3: Participates in physical activity, 3A, 3B, 3C
- Standard 4: Achieves health-enhancing physical fitness, 4A, 4B, 4C, 4D, 4E
- Standard 5: Exhibits responsible behavior and respect for others, 5A, 5B, 5C, 5G, 5H
- Standard 6: Values physical activity for health, and social interactions, 6A, 6B, 6C, 6G

## Week 1 Math Standards

For specific focal points, see appendix B.

- Numbers and operations (counting with understanding, ordinal and cardinal numbers)
- Algebra (sort, classify, order, sequence, pattern, add, subtract)
- Measurement (measurement units, select units and tools, measure in units using measurement tools)
- Data analysis and probability (represent data using concrete objects, pictures, and graphs)

## Week 1 Standards for Other Curriculum Areas

Standards for other academic areas, such as sciences and language arts, were considered in developing lessons. Appendix B includes the sources of these standards.

## Week 1 Resources

There are three types of printed resources for use in Wellness Week 1: signs, worksheets, and newsletters. Web-based resources are also provided.

### Signs

General signs (described in more detail on page 17) can be used during Wellness Week 1 and

reused in subsequent Wellness Weeks. Other signs are specifically for use during Wellness Week 1.

 **General**

G1: Fitness for Life: Elementary School

G2: Wellness Week

G3: Physical Activity Pyramid for Kids

G4: MyPyramid for Kids

G5: Eat Well Wednesday

G6: TEAM Time: Together Everyone Achieves More

G7: Get Fit Friday

G8: Healthy mind, healthy body, healthy heart . . . let's start!

G9: ABCs of Physical Activity

G10: ABCs of Nutrition

 **Wellness Week 1 → Signs**

\*1.1: Be active your way every day!

1.2: Move your muscles when you work and play!

\*1.3: Keep on trying. The more you try, the better you get!

1.4: Green is for veggies, red is for fruits!

\*1.5: Eat the rainbow way: every color, every day!

\*1.6: Eating 5 to 9 fruits and veggies each day helps my body along the way!

\*1.7: Play safely!

1.8: I can, you can, we all can work together!

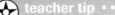

\* Indicates signs used for chants

⭐ **teacher tip** • • •
Choose a bulletin board in your classroom to use for wellness. During each Wellness Week, post the general signs all week. Each day of Wellness Week, feature the signs of the day, or post all daily signs and point out the sign of the day on appropriate days. If possible, feature the sign of the day at the front of the classroom. At the end of Wellness Week, continue to feature wellness on the wellness bulletin board, rotating the signs from time to time.

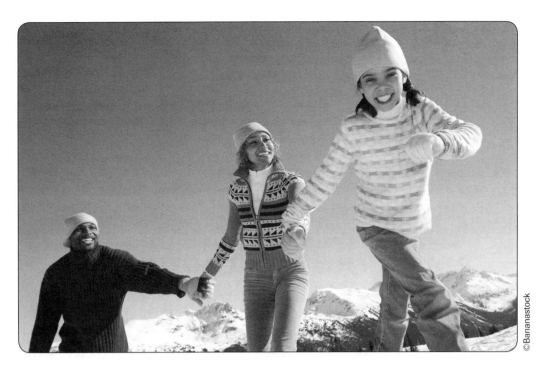

Lessons and messages in Wellness Week 1 emphasize moderate physical activity.

## Worksheets

The DVD includes black-and-white versions of all Week 1 signs that you can print and use as coloring worksheets. In addition, the DVD includes black-and-white versions of MyPyramid for Kids and the Physical Activity Pyramid for Kids for coloring.

 **Wellness Week 1 → Worksheets**

## Newsletters

The DVD contains a newsletter for use during each Wellness Week. It is recommended that your wellness coordinator edit, print, and distribute these newsletters. If you do not have a wellness coordinator, or if your coordinator does not handle the newsletters, you can do it yourself. Just open the appropriate newsletter file, follow the instructions to edit and customize the newsletter, print it, and distribute it, either electronically or by sending copies home with the students. Remind students to talk to their families about Wellness Week and the information in the newsletters.

 **Wellness Week 1 → Newsletter**

## Web Resources

- Available at www.mypyramid.gov: a My-Pyramid worksheet and nutrition activities
- Available at www.dole.com/superkids/: *Kids Cookbook*, games, puzzles, and other nutrition activities

# Week 1 Special Days

Each Wellness Week, two schoolwide activities are featured. On Eat Well Wednesday, nutrition is the focus, and on Get Fit Friday, physical activity is the focus. These activities provide opportunities for the whole school to have a common experience and to highlight the importance of nutrition and physical activity to health and wellness.

## Eat Well Wednesday

During each Wellness Week, Day 3 (typically Wednesday) is known as Eat Well Wednesday. On this day, teachers and staff are encouraged to emphasize the weekly nutrition message. Special schoolwide events (e.g., a lunch salad bar or healthy snack preparation) may be planned by the wellness coordinator. Teachers are encouraged to support these Eat Well Wednesday events and plan special Eat Well Wednesday events in their classrooms, emphasizing sound nutrition. During Wellness Week 1, a special fruit and vegetable bar will be set up in the cafeteria.

## Get Fit Friday

During each Wellness Week, Day 5 (typically Friday) is known as Get Fit Friday. On this day, a schoolwide event focusing on physical activity will be planned by the wellness coordinator. The Get Fit Friday activities are called TEAM Time activities (TEAM stands for Together Everyone Achieves More).

During Wellness Week 1, this activity will be the School Walk. At the designated time, all the students in the school will walk through the halls or walk outside. Your wellness coordinator will provide more information about this activity.

# USING THE VIDEO ACTIVITIES

During each Wellness Week, you will play an activity video every day. The five videos use the same activity routine but present different conceptual messages for each day of the week. Simply play the appropriate video and have your students perform the routine for that day. The DVD also provides an instructional video for each week's routine. If your school has a physical education teacher, he or she may have taught the routine to students during the week before Wellness Week, in which case you won't have to use the instructional video. Otherwise, you can use it to help your students learn the routine.

In the instructional video, the instructor faces away from your students for some of the left–right movements. Explain to students that they should do those movements the same way the instructor does them. That is, when the instructor moves to the right, they should also move to the right. However, in the daily activity videos, the leaders face forward, so their left–right movements are in reverse (mirror image). While following along with the daily activity videos, your students should move in the opposite direction of the leaders for left–right movements. Keep in mind that although moving in the correct direction is desirable, the key is to get all kids moving regardless of the direction. If your students have a hard time performing the activity, feel free to replay the instructional video.

# Day 1 Lesson Plan

## OVERVIEW

✴ **Morning Activity Break**: Get Fit (DVD routine)
✴ **Afternoon Activity Break**: Head, Shoulders, Knees, and Toes

## OBJECTIVES

Students will

✴ participate in 10 minutes of moderate to vigorous physical activity;

✴ repeat the message that physical activity is good for them and fun to do;

✴ list two jobs in which workers are physically active; and

✴ participate in physical activity, making only supportive comments to themselves and others.

## RESOURCES

### Signs

 **General**

G2: Wellness Week

G3: Physical Activity Pyramid for Kids

G8: Healthy mind, healthy body, healthy heart . . . let's start!

 **Wellness Week 1 → Signs**

\* 1.1: Be active your way every day!

1.2: Move your muscles when you work and play!

_____
\* Indicates sign used for chant

### Worksheets

The DVD includes black-and-white versions of today's signs that you can print and use as coloring worksheets. In addition, the DVD includes black-and-white versions of MyPyramid for Kids and the Physical Activity Pyramid for Kids for coloring.

> **teacher tip** • • •
> Your enthusiasm will go a long way to "sell" physical activity as an important part of daily life. Focus on enjoying this active time yourself as well as on the importance of it for your children's minds and bodies! Emphasize moderate activity (the weekly theme) such as walking.

 **Wellness Week 1 → Worksheets**

# MORNING ACTIVITY BREAK

**DVD Routine**: Get Fit

## Introduction

"It's important to be physically active every day. This week we're going to be talking about moderate physical activity. Moderate physical activity includes things we might do as part of our regular day, like walking or working around our houses or in a garden. We may not breathe hard or have our hearts beating really fast when doing moderate physical activity, but it is still good for us. Some people do lots of physical activity as part of their jobs. Can you think of some things workers have to do every day as part of their jobs or regular life?"

Solicit answers and perhaps write them on board, or have the children all act out a couple of suggestions.

Talk with the children about personal space and have them explore the space around them where they can move without touching anyone else. Remind them that they will be moving in their personal space (not around the room) during the movement activities.

**?** **comprehension check** • • •

"Before we start, let's go over a special signal. When I clap my hands like this"—clap your hands three times, or choose your own attention signal—"I want you to stop moving and look at me. Let's practice. Start marching in place. (Clap, clap, clap.) Great job stopping and looking right at me."

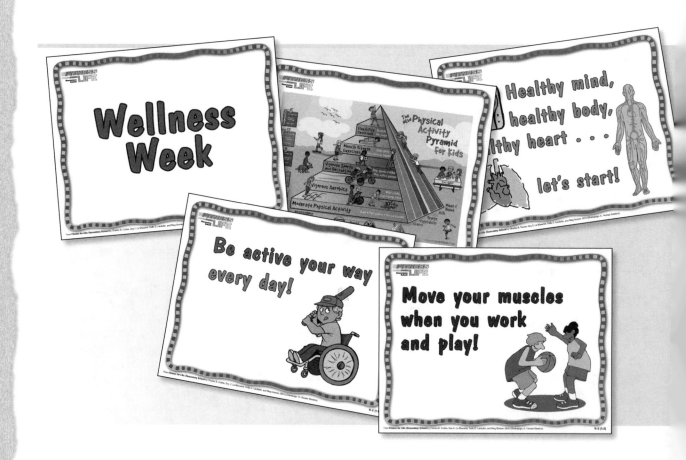

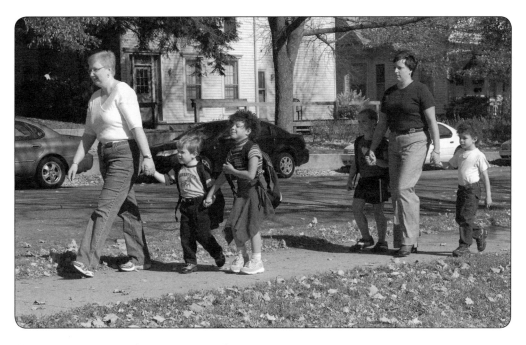

Walking is one way to be active every day.

## Video Routine

The DVD has five versions of the Get Fit routine, one for each day of the week. It also has a special instructional version that teaches students how to do the routine.

1. Play the instructional routine. If the PE teacher has already taught the routine to the students, you can skip this step.
2. Play the Day 1 routine.

Each day the current version of the routine promotes a new and different message. Variations on the message play before the first routine, between routines, and after the last routine. For Get Fit, the Day 1 message is "Be active every day," and the three variations are as follows:

* Move your muscles every day when you work and when you play.
* Walking, playing, slow or fast—being active is a blast.
* Move your body 60 minutes a day; that's an hour for fun and play. Be as active as you can be; play or walk with your family.

## Breathing

After finishing the routine, lead the class in breathing.

"Breathing deeply is important for our bodies, so we'll end every activity with a couple of deep breaths. Let's all breathe in deeply (count 1, 2), hold (count 1, 2), breathe out (count 1, 2), and hold (count 1, 2)." Repeat three times.

## Background Information

* U.S. Department of Health and Human Services activity guidelines (2008) recommend 60 minutes or more of physical activity each day for children and adolescents.

✳ The Physical Activity Pyramid for Kids shows different types of activity. Moderate lifestyle activity provides a great deal of our daily activity.

✳ Either moderate activity (such as walking to school) or vigorous play activity can be used to meet national 60 minute guidelines.

✳ Studies show that children who are active at home (with family) are more likely to meet guidelines than those who are not.

## Discussion

✳ "Raise your hand if you do some activity every day as part of your daily life" (e.g., walk to school, walk the dog, carry a backpack).

✳ "In what kind of jobs do people get exercise?"

✳ "In what kind of jobs do people not get much exercise?"

✳ "Do people in your family have jobs where they do physical activity? What are those jobs?"

✳ "What types of activity do you do every day? What are some physical activities you like to do outside? Inside?"

✳ "Whom do you like to be active with at home?"

## Chant

Chanting is a great way to reinforce messages. If you've posted the corresponding sign, point to it, and tell the students that when you say the first phrase, they should respond by saying the second phrase. Make it fun!

Teacher: "Be active your way . . ."

Students: ". . . every day!"

Practice several times until the students respond easily to your prompt.

## Closure

Closure provides an opportunity to focus one more time on the main message of the lesson by using compliments, reviewing messages, and making suggestions for doing activity at home. Closure also includes a brief preview of what's coming in the next lesson to help students see connections and begin to prepare for future lessons.

### *Compliments*

"You did a great job following the video and got some exercise. It was fun to do this with you."

↻ review • • •

"Today we talked about it being important to do some physical activity every day, and some of you shared things that you like to do outside and inside like . . ." (Here point out activities the students volunteered earlier.)

### *Take It Home*

"Since we all need to get 60 minutes of physical activity every day, maybe you can get someone at home to take a walk with you tonight or do some other physical activity."

### *Preview*

"Since this is Wellness Week, we're really going to try to be especially active. We're going to take a break like this every day."

# AFTERNOON ACTIVITY BREAK

**Activity**: Head, Shoulders, Knees, and Toes

Perform in the afternoon or at some other time during the day when the students need a physical activity break. Teach children the song and motions (touch each body part as you sing it) to "Head, Shoulders, Knees, and Toes":

* ✶ "Head, shoulders, knees, and toes, knees and toes,"
* ✶ "Head, shoulders, knees, and toes, knees and toes,"
* ✶ "Eyes and ears and mouth and nose,"
* ✶ "Head, shoulders, knees, and toes, knees and toes."

After the students understand the activity, challenge them to perform it a little faster. Change some of the words to other body parts and sing again (e.g., "Head, shoulders, thighs and shins, thighs and shins . . . Eyes and ears and mouth and chin . . .").

 **comprehension check** • • •
"Point to your movement space. That's right, move in just one place, not around the room."

## Breathing

After finishing the activity, lead the class in breathing.

"Breathing deeply is important for our bodies, so we'll end every activity with a couple of deep breaths. Let's all breathe in deeply (count 1, 2), hold (count 1, 2), breathe out (count 1, 2), and hold (count 1, 2)." Repeat three times.

## Closure

"Thanks for showing such good body control. You all did that without any problems even though we are in a small space. Since you have such good body control, we'll be able to do lots of fun things because I won't have to worry about you getting hurt when you are moving in this little space."

# ADDITIONAL ACTIVITIES

See appendix A for additional enriching and integrative outdoor activities. For more information, go to www.fitnessforlife.org.

# 1 WELLNESS WEEK

## Day 2 Lesson Plan

### OVERVIEW

* **Morning Activity Break**: Get Fit (DVD routine)
* **Afternoon Activity Break**: Pattern Practice

### OBJECTIVES

Students will

* participate in 10 minutes of moderate to vigorous physical activity;
* when asked, repeat the message that it is important to keep on trying;
* identify a time when they kept on trying to learn something new;
* participate in physical activity, making only supportive comments to themselves and others; and
* identify the correct movement to continue an ABAB pattern and perform the pattern of movements.

### RESOURCES

#### Signs

 **Wellness Week 1 → Signs**

    * 1.3: Keep on trying. The more you try, the better you get!

———————

* Indicates sign used for chant

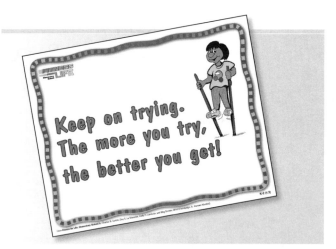

Keep on trying. The more you try, the better you get!

#### Worksheets

The DVD includes a black-and-white version of today's sign that you can print and use as a coloring worksheet. In addition, the DVD includes black-and-white versions of MyPyramid for Kids and the Physical Activity Pyramid for Kids for coloring.

 **Wellness Week 1 → Worksheets**

# MORNING ACTIVITY BREAK

**DVD Routine**: Get Fit

## Introduction

"Yesterday we talked about how important it is to be physically active every day. This week we are talking about moderate physical activity. When we do moderate physical activity, we are being active, but not so active that we are getting really sweaty. To learn new things, we have to try them. Can you think of something that you didn't know how to do, and then after you tried it, you were able to do it?"

Solicit answers from students.

"Today we're going to do the routine with the video again. Since we already did it once, it will be a little easier to do today. We're getting better at it because we are doing it again. Yesterday you all showed me good body control. You were in control of your body and did not bump anyone else. That's great—it kept everyone safe. I'm watching today to see some good body control again."

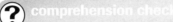 **comprehension check** • • •
"Point to your movement space. That's right, move in just one place, not around the room."

## Video Routine

The DVD has five versions of the Get Fit routine, one for each day of the week. It also has a special instructional version that teaches students how to do the routine.

1. If the students have not done this week's routine before, play the instructional routine. If the PE teacher has already taught the routine to the students, or if they have already practiced the instructional routine with you, you can skip this step.

2. Play the Day 2 routine.

Each day the current version of the routine promotes a new and different message. Variations on the message play before the first routine, between routines, and after the last routine. For Get Fit, the Day 2 message is "Keep on trying," and the three variations are as follows:

✱ The more you try, the better you get. We all can try, you bet, you bet.

✱ It takes more than one try to get good. Try again—I knew you could.

✱ Practice means trying again and again until you get better. So whether you hike, bike, or climb, practice helps you get better every time.

## Breathing

After finishing the routine, lead the class in breathing.

"Breathing deeply is important for our bodies, so we'll end every activity with a couple of deep breaths. Let's all breathe in deeply (count 1, 2), hold (count 1, 2), breathe out (count 1, 2), and hold (count 1, 2)." Repeat three times.

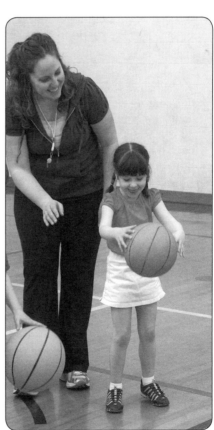

To improve any physical activity skill, you have to keep on trying.

WEEK 1 • DAY 2

## Background Information

* When learning motor skills, you never know at what point you are going to "get" something. Always give it one more try.
* When practicing new skills, begin with simple tasks or versions of the activity, and then move to more complex tasks or versions of the activity.
* Make trying and practice fun. Do it with a friend!
* Practicing a little each day is usually better than practicing all at one time.

## Discussion

* "Do you think people ever have to try new things at their jobs? If someone said, 'I don't know how to do that, so I won't try,' what do you think would happen?"
* "Have you ever tried something new that you hadn't done before? Did you start slowly? Was it a little scary to try it because you hadn't ever done it before? How did it turn out?"
* "Can you remember something you were a little scared to try, but when you tried it, you really liked it?"
* "Do you think it is better to practice for a long time one day or to practice a little bit every day?"

## Chant

Chanting is a great way to reinforce messages. If you've posted the corresponding sign, point to it, and tell the students that when you say the first phrase, they should respond by saying the second phrase. Make it fun!

> ⊛ **teacher tip** • • •
> Chanting can be fun and really help remind us of important points. Be enthusiastic, use different accents, and sometimes allow the students to shout back their response. Encourage students to teach the chants to their families.

Teacher: "Keep on trying. The more you try . . ."

Students: ". . . the better you get!"

Practice several times until the students respond easily to your prompt.

## Closure

Closure provides an opportunity to focus one more time on the main message of the lesson by using compliments, reviewing messages, and making suggestions for doing activity at home. Closure also includes a brief preview of what's coming in the next lesson to help students see connections and begin to prepare for future lessons.

### Compliments

"You did a great job following the video, and I can see you are getting better at it because you are practicing. Practice helps us get better at things."

> ↻ **review** • • •
> "Today we talked a lot about practice and how it helps us get better. How can you tell when you are getting better at something? What does it feel like?"

### Take It Home

"When you are at home, think about what would be good things to try—perhaps new food? Try to eat fruits and veggies that you never have eaten before and tell us about it when you come to school!"

### Preview

"Tomorrow we will practice moving with the video again."

# AFTERNOON ACTIVITY BREAK

**Activity**: Pattern Practice

Perform in the afternoon or at other times when the students need a physical activity break.

"A pattern is something you repeat over and over in the same way. Here is a letter pattern: A B A B A B A. What do you think comes next? Yes, B. OK, let's try a stand up, sit down pattern. Stand up, sit down, stand up, sit down, stand up, sit down, stand up. What's next? Right, sit down. Let's do another pattern. How about reach up high, put your hands on your hips, reach high, hands on hips, reach high, hands on hips. Who can think of another pattern to do?" Write the pattern on the board.

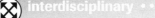

**interdisciplinary** • • •
This activity helps students practice patterns in movement. Being able to recognize, follow, and create patterns are also important skills in math.

Talk about patterns, about how to extend them, and about how you can look at them in different ways: as single units, as groups of units (eg., A B A B = AB AB), and so on.

## Breathing

After finishing the activity, lead the class in breathing.

"Breathing deeply is important for our bodies, so we'll end every activity with a couple of deep breaths. Let's all breathe in deeply (count 1, 2), hold (count 1, 2), breathe out (count 1, 2), and hold (count 1, 2)." Repeat three times.

**observation** • • •
Look around the room. Are the children showing good body control? Are they easily following the pattern? If someone is having trouble, try using easier combinations, such as having both hands do the same thing. If the movements seem easy for everyone, and children are getting bored, choose some more complex actions to incorporate (e.g., hopping on one side and then the other, using one arm and then the other).

## Closure

"Thanks for showing such good body control. You all did that without any problems even though we are in a small space. Since you have such good body control, we can keep doing active games in the classroom. I won't have to worry about you getting hurt when you are moving in this little space."

# ADDITIONAL ACTIVITIES

See appendix A for additional enriching and integrative outdoor activities. For more information, go to www.fitnessforlife.org.

WEEK 1 • DAY 2

# 1 WELLNESS WEEK

## Day 3 Lesson Plan

### OVERVIEW

* **Morning Activity Break**: Get Fit (DVD routine)
* **Eat Well Wednesday Class Discussion**: Track Your Fruits and Veggies
* **Eat Well Wednesday Activity**: A to Z Fruit and Veggie Bar in the Cafeteria
* **Afternoon Activity Break**: Simon Says

### OBJECTIVES

Students will

* participate in 10 minutes of moderate to vigorous physical activity,
* repeat (correctly) the message that daily physical activity is important for health and fun to do,
* name fruits and veggies of at least three different colors,
* practice decision making and attention by responding with movement on appropriate verbal cues (Simon Says) and not responding when the cue is missing,
* identify the color of the fruit and vegetable stripes on the food pyramid (green = veggies, red = fruits), and
* identify that vitamins come from plants, animals, and the sun.

### RESOURCES

#### Signs

 **General**

> G4: MyPyramid for Kids
>
> G5: Eat Well Wednesday
>
> G10: ABCs of Nutrition

 **Wellness Week 1 → Signs**

> 1.4: Green is for veggies, red is for fruits!
>
> * 1.5: Eat the rainbow way: every color, every day!
>
> * 1.6: Eating 5 to 9 fruits and veggies each day helps my body along the way!

---

\* Indicates signs used for chants

## Worksheets

The DVD includes black-and-white versions of today's signs that you can print and use as coloring worksheets. In addition, the DVD includes black-and-white versions of MyPyramid for Kids and the Physical Activity Pyramid for Kids for coloring.

 **Wellness Week 1 → Worksheets**

## Web Resources

> Available at www.mypyramid.gov: With the help of a parent or family member, students can keep track of what they eat using MyTracker.

# MORNING ACTIVITY BREAK

**DVD Routine**: Get Fit

## Introduction

"Being physically active every day is great. Yesterday we talked about how important it is to keep trying when we are learning new activities. To have enough energy to be active, we need to eat healthy foods. Eating fruits gives us energy. We're going to do our video routine again. It should be easier today because this is our third day trying it. Show me your good body control again today."

## Video Routine

The DVD has five versions of the Get Fit routine, one for each day of the week. It also has a special instructional version that teaches students how to do the routine.

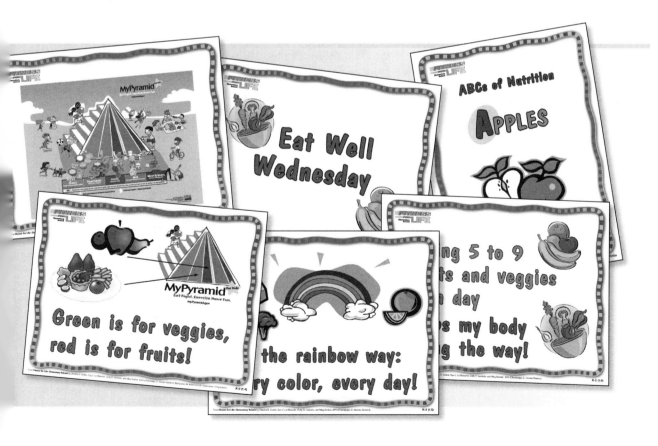

WEEK 1 · DAY 3

1. If the students have not done this week's routine before, play the instructional routine. If the PE teacher has already taught the routine to the students, or if they have already practiced the instructional routine with you, you can skip this step.

2. Play the Day 3 routine.

Each day the current version of the routine promotes a new and different message. Variations on the message play before the first the routine, between routines, and after the last routine. For Get Fit, the Day 3 message is "Fitness foods," and the three variations are as follows:

* Fruits have colors of the rainbow and give you energy to help you grow.
* Veggies have colors of the rainbow and give you energy to help you grow.
* Rainbow-colored foods are good to eat. Red strawberries, green veggies, orange carrots, and blueberries are a special treat.

**observation** • • •
Look around the room. Are the children showing good body control? Are there any parts of the routine that are particularly hard, creating stumbling blocks for the students? Note any difficult parts so you can either have the students practice that piece or modify the routine to allow them to flow through it.

## Breathing

After finishing the routine, lead the class in breathing.

"Breathing deeply is important for our bodies, so we'll end every activity with a couple of deep breaths. Let's all breathe in deeply (count 1, 2), hold (count 1, 2), breathe out (count 1, 2), and hold (count 1, 2)." Repeat three times.

## Background Information

* The color of a fruit or vegetable often indicates the type of nutrient found in it. Eating lots of colors means you get all the different nutrients.
* The U.S. Department of Agriculture recommends that people consume a variety of fruits and vegetables each day for health.
* The U.S. Department of Agriculture states that eating a diet rich in fruits and vegetables may reduce the risk for type 2 diabetes.
* Eat 5 to 9 servings of fruit and vegetables each day.

## Discussion

* "Raise your hand if you can think of a red fruit or veggie? How about an orange one?"
* "What other fruits can you think of that are other colors?"
* "Let's make a list of fruits you eat a lot. It's good to eat at least four (or five) fruits and veggies every day. Let's think of five fruits and veggies." (Answers might include bananas, raisins, apples, carrots, or blueberries.)
* "Use the alphabet to list fruits and veggies from A to Z. Try to get one for each letter."

## Chant

Chanting is a great way to reinforce messages. If you've posted the corresponding sign, point to it, and tell the students that when you say the first phrase, they should respond by saying the second phrase. Make it fun!

Teacher: "Eat the rainbow way . . ."

Students: ". . . every color, every day!"

Teacher: "Eating 5 to 9 fruits and veggies each day . . ."

Students: ". . . helps my body along the way!"

Practice several times until the students respond easily to your prompt.

## Closure

Closure provides an opportunity to focus one more time on the main message of the lesson by using compliments, reviewing messages, and making suggestions for doing activity at home. Closure also includes a brief preview of what's coming in the next lesson to help students see connections and begin to prepare for future lessons.

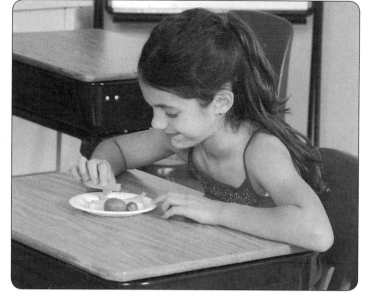

Fruits and veggies are fitness foods that provide energy.

### *Compliments*

"You make this routine look easy. Trying it each day has helped us get better."

### *Take It Home*

"Help the person who shops for food at your house know what

**⟳ review** • • •

"Show me with your fingers how many fruits and veggies you should eat each day. Think about the colors of your favorite fruits and veggies."

fruits and veggies you like. How could you tell them? Let's practice what you might say."

### *Preview*

"Tomorrow we're going to be talking about safety and movement."

# EAT WELL WEDNESDAY

Each Wednesday all teachers and staff are encouraged to emphasize the weekly nutrition message. Special schoolwide events (e.g., a lunch salad bar or healthy snack preparation) may be planned by the wellness coordinator. Teachers are encouraged to support these Eat Well Wednesday events and plan special Eat Well Wednesday events in their classrooms, emphasizing sound nutrition.

## Eat Well Wednesday Class Discussion

**Nutrition Topic:** Track Your Fruits and Veggies

### *Introduction*

Introduce MyPyramid and the healthy food group of the week—fruits and vegetables. MyPyramid is a nutrition guideline used to promote healthy eating and to introduce the five food groups (plus oils): grains, vegetables, fruits, milk, and meat and beans. Each food group represents a different nutritional category.

### *Background Information*

* When you treat your body well, it will grow, keep itself strong, and heal itself when hurt.

* Nutrients are elements in healthy foods with special jobs. There are six nutrient types (carbohydrate, vitamins, minerals, fat, protein, and water).

* By eating a wide variety of foods our bodies receive all the nutrients they need to learn, move, and grow.

* Fruits and vegetables provide us with the vitamins and minerals our bodies needs.

* Vitamins are elements from plants, animals, or the sun, like vitamin D. Minerals are elements from the soil like iron, copper, and zinc.

* Different colors of foods have different vitamins and minerals. Good nutrition means eating for good health. This week our challenge will be to eat a wide variety of fruits and vegetables so our body receives all the nutrients it needs to learn, move, and grow!

### Discussion

* "What are some reasons fruits and vegetables are important to your body?"

* "How many minutes of activity did you do yesterday? Did you get 60 minutes of physical activity yesterday?"

* "How many fruits did you eat yesterday? How many vegetables? Did you eat your 5 to 9 fruits and vegetables yesterday? That means at least 5 fruits and veggies every day, and you can eat more than 5—up to 9. Let's count up how many I had yesterday." Name and count your fruits and veggies from the day before.

> **review** • • •
> • "What is MyPyramid?"
> • "Turn to your neighbors and tell them your favorite vegetable or fruit."
> • "Turn to your neighbors and name an orange, green, red, yellow, blue, or purple fruit or vegetable."

### Take It Home

* "Find out a family member's favorite vegetable or fruit."

* "Go shopping with your family and buy one new fruit or vegetable."

* "Tell your parents or guardians what fruits and veggies you like best."

* "Ask if you can have a fruit or veggie snack at home."

## Eat Well Wednesday Schoolwide Activity

During Wellness Week 1, a special fruit and vegetable bar will be set up in the cafeteria.

# AFTERNOON ACTIVITY BREAK

**Activity**: Simon Says

Perform in the afternoon or at some other time during the day when the students need a physical activity break.

> **interdisciplinary** • • •
> This activity includes movement and helps students practice categorizing skills since they have to put the instructions into one of two categories: instructions to follow and instructions to ignore. The activity also provides practice in number operations by using various methods for defining the number of times to do each movement.

Begin by explaining how the game works. Tell them that when you start an instruction with "Simon says," they should do what you say. But if you simply tell them to do something, such as "Wave your arms," they shouldn't respond. Then lead them through several examples so they understand how the game works. For instance, if you say, "Simon says, 'Put your hands on your hips,'" the students should put their hands on their hips. But if you say, "Put your hands on your hips," the students should not do it.

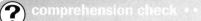
**comprehension check** • • •
Ask the students to show you what they will do if you say, "Simon says, 'Touch your shoulders.'" Ask what they will do if you say, "Touch your knees" without saying, "Simon says" first.

If students make mistakes just say "oops," laugh with them, and go on with the next action. Suggested actions:

* Stand up.
* Sit down.
* Jump or march or run in place so many number of times.
* Make a shape like a banana, apple, orange, or pineapple.
* Put your hands on your head, shoulders, knees, toes, elbows, or thighs.
* Turn around.
* Do daily living actions, such as walk to school, pretend to get a book off a shelf, stir food, or sweep the floor.

Use number operations when telling the students the number of times to do something (e.g., instead of telling them four times, use two plus two). Have students use addition, subtraction, less than, more than, and so on to determine the number of times to do each exercise. Reinforce vocabulary about the relative position and the magnitude of ordinal and cardinal numbers.

## Breathing

After finishing the activity, lead the class in breathing.

"Breathing deeply is important for our bodies so we'll end every activity with a couple of deep breaths. Let's all breathe in deeply (count 1, 2), hold (count 1, 2), breathe out (count 1, 2), and hold (count 1, 2)." Repeat three times.

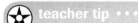
**teacher tip** • • •
Try to make discussions about foods empowering for children. Focus on the foods that will help build their bodies and celebrate the enjoyment and empowerment associated with choosing nutritious foods.

## Closure

"Thanks for showing such good body control. You paid careful attention to what Simon said to do. That's careful listening. Careful listening helps you learn lots of new things."

# ADDITIONAL ACTIVITIES

See appendix A for additional enriching and integrative outdoor activities. For more information, go to www.fitnessforlife.org.

# 1 WELLNESS WEEK

## Day 4 Lesson Plan

### OVERVIEW

* **Morning Activity Break**: Get Fit (DVD routine)
* **Afternoon Activity Break**: Follow the Leader

### OBJECTIVES

Students will

* participate in 10 minutes of moderate to vigorous physical activity;
* identify two kinds of safety equipment that are important to keep them safe;
* list at least one kind of safety equipment that they should wear when being active;
* participate in physical activity, making only supportive comments to themselves and others; and
* count steps.

### RESOURCES

#### Signs

 **Wellness Week 1 → Signs**

  \* 1.7: Play safely!

\* Indicates sign used for chant

#### Worksheets

The DVD includes a black-and-white version of today's sign that you can print and use as a coloring worksheet. In addition, the DVD includes black-and-white versions of MyPyramid for Kids and the Physical Activity Pyramid for Kids for coloring.

 **Wellness Week 1 → Worksheets**

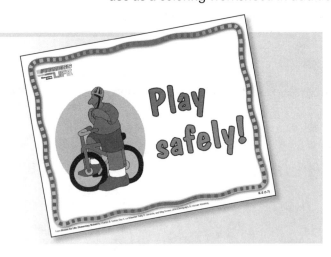

### MORNING ACTIVITY BREAK

**DVD Routine**: Get Fit

#### Introduction

"Yesterday we talked about what good, healthy foods fruits and veggies are. They give us energy to move. When we move, good body control helps keep us safe. Sometimes we need to protect our bodies with special equipment like helmets. I wonder what safety equipment people use in their jobs. What safety equipment do you use?"

Solicit ideas like bike helmets and pads.

"We should be able to do the routine today without even thinking about it, since we've been practicing it all week. Let's see what we remember. It's OK to sing along."

## Video Routine

The DVD has five versions of the Get Fit routine, one for each day of the week. It also has a special instructional version that teaches students how to do the routine.

1. If the students have not done this week's routine before, play the instructional routine. If the PE teacher has already taught the routine to the students, or if they have already practiced the instructional routine with you, you can skip this step.

2. Play the Day 4 routine.

Each day the current version of the routine promotes a new and different message. Variations on the message play before the first routine, between routines, and after the last routine. For Get Fit, the Day 4 message is "Play safely," and the three variations are as follows:

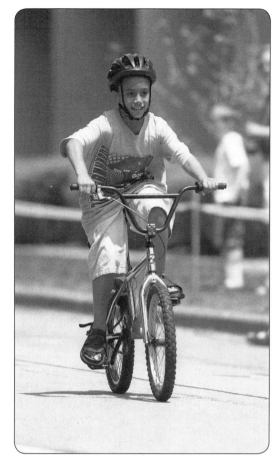

For safe play, wear a helmet and other special equipment.

✳ Wear helmets, pads, sunscreen, and shoes. Playing safe is what we choose.

✳ Helmets for heads and hats for sun; playing safe is much more fun.

✳ Playing is much more fun when no one gets hurt. Equipment can help keep you safe, but safety starts with you. Use your ears to listen to instructions about playing safely, and use your eyes to spot danger during play.

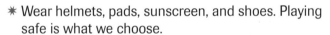

**observation** • • •
Look around the room. Are the students doing the activity with ease? Tell them how well they are doing and how much better they have gotten with practice.

## Breathing

After finishing the routine, lead the class in breathing.

"Breathing deeply is important for our bodies, so we'll end every activity with a couple of deep breaths. Let's all breathe in deeply (count 1, 2), hold (count 1, 2), breathe out (count 1, 2), and hold (count 1, 2)." Repeat three times.

## Background Information

✳ Your brain is soft and cushioned inside your skull. Helmets help make sure that it doesn't get bruised if you hit your head. Bruises on your brain can make it difficult to think and talk.

✳ Sunscreen protects your skin from the rays of the sun that can burn your skin and can cause skin cancer.

WEEK 1 • DAY 4

✳ Good playing shoes help prevent blisters and provide a cushion for your foot. Since the weight of your body comes down on your foot, it is nice to have a cushion under it.

✳ Good playing shoes stay on your feet so your feet are protected.

## Discussion

✳ "What should you wear on your head when you ride a bike?"

✳ "What other activities use helmets?"

✳ "Are there other kinds of equipment that protect you when you are active?"

✳ "How can we help people remember to put on their helmets?"

✳ "How can listening to your teacher or family help you be safe?"

## Chant

Chanting is a great way to reinforce messages. If you've posted the corresponding sign, point to it, and tell the students that when you say the first phrase, they should respond by saying the second phrase. Make it fun!

Teacher: "Play . . ."

Students: ". . . safely!"

Practice several times until the students respond easily to your prompt.

## Closure

Closure provides an opportunity to focus one more time on the main message of the lesson by using compliments, reviewing messages, and making suggestions for doing activity at home. Closure also includes a brief preview of what's coming in the next lesson to help students see connections and begin to prepare for future lessons.

↺ **review** • • •

"So far this week we've talked about making physical activity a part of every day, trying again and again, eating the rainbow of fruits and veggies, and wearing safety equipment. Think about eating your favorite fruit or veggie."

• "Is it crunchy or soft?"

• "Is it rough on the outside, or is it smooth?"

• "Is it sweet or tart?"

### Compliments

"You're getting so good at the routine that you can almost do it without thinking about it. Paying close attention to the leader helps you do it better each day."

### Take It Home

"Help people at your house remember these things every day. You might want to be A PEST at home to remind everyone of these important ideas:

✳ Be **A**ctive every day.

✳ **P**ractice to get better.

✳ **E**at the rainbow way every day.

✳ Play **S**afely.

✳ **T**eamwork always.

"Write the letters A PEST on a sheet of paper so you will remember what the letters mean. Eating right and exercising will help you learn, move, and grow!"

*Preview*

"Tomorrow we'll do Get Fit one more time and use the alphabet to help us get active."

# AFTERNOON ACTIVITY BREAK

**Activity**: Follow the Leader

Perform in the afternoon or at some other time during the day when the students need a physical activity break.

Start with simple actions, having the children follow your actions. Try to do at least 8 counts of each movement—clap your hands, 1, 2, 3, 4, 5, 6, 7, 8; march in place, 1, 2, 3, 4, 5, 6, 7, 8; put your hands in the air and wave them back and forth, 1, 2, 3, 4, 5, 6, 7, 8 (put them down after 8), and so on. Other suggestions you might try are tap your head, shoulders, hips, and toes; bend and straighten knees; lean right, lean left; stretch high; twist right, twist left; or run in place.

Let different students take turns leading. Estimate how many step it is around the classroom, and have students estimate how many steps it is along one side of the room. Discuss steps as units of measurement and why different people will get different answers for their estimates (because of different leg and stride lengths).

## Breathing

After finishing the activity, lead the class in breathing.

"Breathing deeply is important for our bodies, so we'll end every activity with a couple of deep breaths. Let's all breathe in deeply (count 1, 2), hold (count 1, 2), breathe out (count 1, 2), and hold (count 1, 2)." Repeat three times.

## Closure

"Thanks for showing such good body control. Yesterday you paid careful attention to what Simon said. Today you paid careful attention to what I was doing. That takes careful watching. Careful watching helps you learn lots of new things."

# ADDITIONAL ACTIVITIES

See appendix A for additional enriching and integrative outdoor activities. For more information, go to www.fitnessforlife.org.

WEEK 1 • DAY 4

# 1 WELLNESS WEEK

## Day 5 Lesson Plan ••••••••••••••••••••••••••

### OVERVIEW

* **Get Fit Friday Activity**: TEAM Time 1: School Walk
* **Morning Activity Break**: Get Fit (DVD routine)
* **Afternoon Activity Break**: Alphabet Lineup

### OBJECTIVES

Students will

* participate in 10 minutes of moderate to vigorous physical activity;
* move fluidly and confidently during the video routine;
* repeat the message that the secret to success is trying;
* demonstrate understanding of a bar graph by identifying the most common letters of first names;
* participate in physical activity, making only supportive comments to themselves and others; and
* be members of the team who try to help the team accomplish the task (Alphabet Lineup) by using good body control, manners, thinking, and listening to others.

### RESOURCES

#### Signs

 **General**

G6: TEAM Time: Together Everyone Achieves More
G7: Get Fit Friday

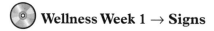 **Wellness Week 1 → Signs**

1.8: I can, you can, we all can work together!

#### Worksheets

The DVD includes a black-and-white version of today's sign that you can print and use as a coloring worksheet. In addition, the DVD includes black-and-white versions of MyPyramid for Kids and the Physical Activity Pyramid for Kids for coloring.

 **Wellness Week 1 → Worksheets**

# GET FIT FRIDAY

During each Wellness Week, Day 5 (typically Friday) is known as Get Fit Friday. On this day, a schoolwide event focusing on physical activity will be planned by the wellness coordinator. The Get Fit Friday activities are called TEAM Time activities (TEAM stands for Together Everyone Achieves More).

During Wellness Week 1, this activity will be the School Walk. At the designated time, all the students in the school will walk through the halls or walk outside. Your wellness coordinator will provide more information about this activity.

In addition to supporting the School Walk, mention the TEAM Time activity as you discuss the video routine messages during the morning activity break.

# MORNING ACTIVITY BREAK

**DVD Routine**: Get Fit

## Introduction

"We've been doing the Get Fit video all week, so today we should be getting pretty good at it. I hope you can sing along as you do it. It is hard at first to do two things at once, like singing and doing the routine, but as you get better at something, you don't need to think about it so much, and you can begin to do two things at once. Try it. Trying hard means paying attention to what you are doing, but when you have done that a lot, and you get really good, sometimes you just do it without even having to think about it. Let's see if we can do this routine well enough to sing at the same time."

## Video Routine

The DVD has five versions of the Get Fit routine, one for each day of the week. It also has a special instructional version that teaches students how to do the routine.

1. If the students have not done this week's routine before, play the instructional routine. If the PE teacher has already taught the routine to the students, or if they have already practiced the instructional routine with you, you can skip this step.

2. Play the Day 5 routine.

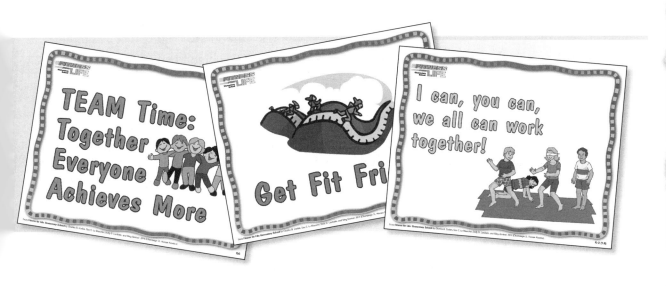

Each day the current version of the routine promotes a new and different message. Variations on the message play before the first routine, between routines, and after the last routine. For Get Fit, the Day 5 message is "I can, you can, we all can," and the three variations are as follows:

✳ I know we can do it; I'll tell you why. We can do it if we try, try, try!

✳ I know we can do it; I'll tell you why. We can do it if we try, try, try!

✳ The secret to success is trying. When you and your teammates try something together, anything is possible. Always give yourself a chance to be successful by trying.

## Breathing

After finishing the routine, lead the class in breathing.

"Breathing deeply is important for our bodies, so we'll end every activity with a couple of deep breaths. Let's all breathe in deeply (count 1, 2), hold (count 1, 2), breathe out (count 1, 2), and hold (count 1, 2)." Repeat three times.

## Background Information

✳ When you and your teammates encourage each other, you help everyone succeed.

✳ Encouragement helps people keep trying.

✳ You don't know what you can do unless you try.

✳ Teamwork makes trying new things fun!

✳ Cooperation means you work together to help reach a goal.

## Discussion

✳ "What would happen if we were on a team trying to do something together, and some people tried, but other people didn't? Would you be able to get the job done?"

✳ "How is everyone trying to make our class better? Can you give an example?" (Answers might include listening when someone else is talking or offering to help carry something.)

✳ "Can you be someone who tries on our class team?"

## Chant

Chanting is a great way to reinforce messages. Use your favorite chants from previous lessons. If you've posted the corresponding sign, point to it, and tell the students that when you say the first phrase, they should respond by saying the second phrase. Make it fun!

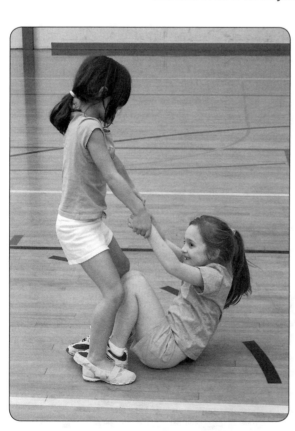

The secret to success is to keep on trying. When teammates try together, anything is possible.

Teacher: "Be active your way . . ."

Students: ". . . every day!"

Teacher: "Keep on trying. The more you try . . ."

Students: ". . . the better you get!"

Teacher: "Eat the rainbow way . . ."

Students: ". . . every color, every day!"

Practice several times until the students respond easily to your prompt.

## Closure

Closure provides an opportunity to focus one more time on the main message of the lesson by using compliments, reviewing messages, and making suggestions for doing activity at home. Closure also includes a brief preview of what's coming in the next lesson to help students see connections and begin to prepare for future lessons.

> **teacher tip • • •**
> "Nice time" refers to taking a few minutes to encourage students to compliment each other on their work. Starting with a stem such as "I'd like to compliment _____ because he did a great job of _____" teaches the students how to identify a particular action to compliment. If you honor this time, the students will, too.

### Compliments

"You're getting so good at the routine that you can almost do it without thinking about it, and I heard you singing along! Practicing something every day helps you get better at it. When you get really good at something, you are able to do two things at one time—sing and move."

### Take It Home

"Have you asked for more fruits and veggies at home? Have you gone for a walk or played with someone at home after school?"

> **review • • •**
> "This week we did the Get Fit routine. We've been talking about moderate activity where you move around some, but not so fast that you get really sweaty. We also talked about fruits and veggies being good things to eat as well as how important it is to use safety equipment and to keep trying when you are learning new things."

### Preview

"During the next Wellness Week, we'll talk about vigorous activity in which you move around so much you get a little sweaty and breathe harder."

## AFTERNOON ACTIVITY BREAK

**Activity**: Alphabet Lineup

Perform in the afternoon or at some other time during the day when the students need a physical activity break.

"We're going to line up in a special way today. I'm going to tell you a way to line up, and I want you to figure out where you should get in line. We're going to use the alphabet. Let's sing it together. When we sing the letter that starts your first name, come get in line. We'll start with As right here and make the line go that way. Ready, A—all the As come line up. B C D E F G H I J K L M N O P Q R S T U V W X Y Z. Let's clap once, jump two times, and march three times. Now let's march around the room in line as we sing the Alphabet Song. Show your good body control by not touching anything as we go."

Use number operations when telling the students the number of times to do something (e.g., instead of "four," say "two plus two"). Have students solve addition and

**interdisciplinary** •••
This activity requires practice in sequencing as well as movement.

subtraction problems to determine the number of times they should do each exercise. Try other operations such as more than and less than. Reinforce vocabulary about the relative position and the magnitude of ordinal and cardinal numbers in talking about position in the line.

## Breathing

After finishing the activity, lead the class in breathing.

"Breathing deeply is important for our bodies, so we'll end every activity with a couple of deep breaths. Let's all breathe in deeply (count 1, 2), hold (count 1, 2), breathe out (count 1, 2), and hold (count 1, 2)." Repeat three times.

## Closure

"You are good listeners and thinkers. Thanks for showing such good body control. On Wednesday, you listened carefully when we played Simon Says. Yesterday you watched carefully and did what I did when we played Follow the Leader. Today you thought carefully about your letter and the alphabet as we lined up."

## ADDITIONAL ACTIVITIES

See appendix A for additional enriching and integrative outdoor activities. For more information, go to www.fitnessforlife.org.

# WELLNESS WEEK

## 2

# Fitness for Life Elementary School

## Week 2 Overview

Table 2.2 is a summary chart of the Wellness Week 2 activities for the second grade classroom. Pages 55 through 78 provide the daily lesson plans for each day of week 2.

- Week 2 physical activity theme: Vigorous physical activity (vigorous aerobics, sports, and recreation)
- Week 2 nutrition theme: Grains and foods with fat

## Week 2 NASPE Standards

Week 2 activities meet the National Association for Sport and Physical Education (NASPE) standards listed here. For full standards and specific performance indicators (e.g., 1A through 6G), see appendix B.

- Standard 1: Motor skills and movement patterns, 1A, 1B, 1C, 1E, 1F
  - Standard 2: Movement concepts and principles, 2C, 2D

**Table 2.2  Summary of Wellness Week 2 Activities**

| Activity | Day 1 Monday | Day 2 Tuesday | Day 3 Wednesday | Day 4 Thursday | Day 5 Friday |
|---|---|---|---|---|---|
| Morning Activity Break | Video routine performed every day of the week: La Raspa | | | | |
| Daily Message | Get your body moving. | Get better with practice. | Foods with fats; grains | Exercise your heart. | Never, ever give up! |
| Afternoon Activity Break | Itsy Bitsy Spider | Pattern Practice | Simon Says | Follow the Leader | Shirt Color Lineup |
| Eat Well Wednesday Classroom Discussion | — | — | Whole Grains and Breakfast | — | — |
| Schoolwide Events | — | — | Eat Well Wednesday: Healthy Breakfast Promotion | — | Get Fit Friday: TEAM Time 2: Big Kids Lead |

- Standard 3: Participates in physical activity, 3A, 3B, 3C
- Standard 4: Achieves health-enhancing physical fitness, 4A, 4B, 4C, 4E
- Standard 5: Exhibits responsible behavior and respect for others, 5A, 5B, 5C, 5G
- Standard 6: Values physical activity for health and social interaction, 6A, 6B, 6C, 6G

## Week 2 Math Standards

For specific focal points see appendix B.

- Numbers and operations (counting with understanding, ordinal and cardinal numbers)
- Algebra (sort, classify, order, sequence, pattern, add, subtract)
- Measurement (measure units, select units and tools, measure in units using measurement tools)
- Data analysis and probability (represent data using concrete objects, pictures, and graphs)

## Week 2 Standards for Other Curriculum Areas

Standards for other academic areas, such as sciences and language arts, were considered in developing lessons. Appendix B includes the sources of these standards.

## Week 2 Resources

There are three types of printed resources for use in Wellness Week 2: signs, worksheets, and newsletters. Web-based resources are also provided.

### Signs

General signs (described in more detail on page 17) can be used during Wellness Week 2 and reused in subsequent Wellness Weeks. Other signs are specifically for use during Wellness Week 2.

 **General**

G1: Fitness for Life: Elementary School

G2: Wellness Week

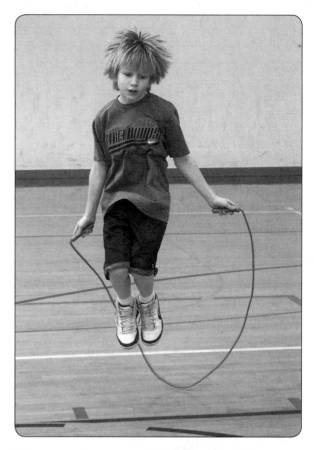

Lessons and messages in Wellness Week 2 emphasize vigorous physical activity.

G3: Physical Activity Pyramid for Kids

G4: MyPyramid for Kids

G5: Eat Well Wednesday

G6: TEAM Time: Together Everyone Achieves More

G7: Get Fit Friday

G8: Healthy mind, healthy body, healthy heart . . . let's start!

G9: ABCs of Physical Activity

G10: ABCs of Nutrition

 **Wellness Week 2 → Signs**

2.1: Physical Activity Pyramid: Make some activity vigorous!

2.2: Get your body moving!

*2.3: Being active is a great start! Being active builds my heart!

*2.4: If it makes you breathe hard and sweat, it helps your brain and body, you bet!

\*2.5: The more you practice, the better you play; practice, practice every day!

2.6: Orange is for grains!

2.7: Make half your grains whole!

2.8: Avoid empty calories!

\*2.9: Some fats are good, some fats are bad. What kind of fats has your body had?

2.10: Break the fast with breakfast!

2.11: Making your heart beat fast helps your body last!

2.12: A healthy heart is a happy heart!

\*2.13: Exercising your heart daily really pays. Your heart will thank you in many ways!

\*2.14: Keep on going to get fit. Never give up! Never quit!

———————————

\* Indicates signs used for chants

> ⭐ **teacher tip** • • •
> Choose a bulletin board to use for wellness in your classroom. During each Wellness Week, post the general signs all week. Each day of Wellness Week, feature the signs of the day, or post all daily signs and point out the sign of the day on appropriate days. If possible, feature the sign of the day at the front of the classroom. At the end of Wellness Week, continue to feature wellness on the wellness bulletin board, rotating signs from time to time.

## Worksheets

The DVD includes black-and-white versions of all Week 2 signs that you can print and use as coloring worksheets. In addition, the DVD includes black-and-white versions of MyPyramid for Kids and the Physical Activity Pyramid for Kids for coloring.

 **Wellness Week 2 → Worksheets**

## Newsletters

The DVD contains a newsletter for use during each Wellness Week. It is recommended that your wellness coordinator edit, print, and distribute these newsletters. If you do not have a wellness coordinator, or if your coordinator does not handle the newsletters, you can do it yourself. Just open the appropriate newsletter file, follow the instructions to edit and customize the newslet-

ter, print it, and distribute it, either electronically or by sending copies home with the students. Remind students to talk to their families about Wellness Week and the information in the newsletters.

 **Wellness Week 2 → Newsletter**

## Web Resources

Available at www.mypyramid.gov: A MyPyramid worksheet and nutrition activities

Available at www.dole.com/superkids/: *Kids Cookbook*, games, puzzles, and other nutrition activities

# Week 2 Special Days

Each Wellness Week, two schoolwide activities are featured. On Eat Well Wednesday, nutrition is the focus, and on Get Fit Friday, physical activity is the focus. These activities provide opportunities for the whole school to have a common experience and to highlight the importance of nutrition and physical activity to health and wellness.

## Eat Well Wednesday

During each Wellness Week, Day 3 (typically Wednesday) is known as Eat Well Wednesday. On this day, teachers and staff are encouraged to emphasize the weekly nutrition message. Special schoolwide events (e.g., a lunch salad bar or healthy snack preparation) may be planned by the wellness coordinator. Teachers are encouraged to support these Eat Well Wednesday events and plan special Eat Well Wednesday events in their classrooms, emphasizing sound nutrition. During Wellness Week 2, healthy breakfasts will be featured in the cafeteria.

## Get Fit Friday

During each Wellness Week, Day 5 (typically Friday) is known as Get Fit Friday. On this day, a schoolwide event focusing on physical activity will be planned by the wellness coordinator. The Get Fit Friday activities are called TEAM Time activities (TEAM stands for Together Everyone Achieves More).

During Wellness Week 2, the TEAM Time activity planned for Get Fit Friday is called Big Kids Lead. The wellness coordinator will lead the activity at the beginning of the school day with the help of students in fifth and sixth grades. All students in the school will congregate outside or in the gym or multipurpose room so that they all can participate together. The TEAM Time activity includes a warm-up, a special routine called Colors, and a cool-down.

# USING THE VIDEO ACTIVITIES

During each Wellness Week, you will play an activity video every day. The five videos use the same activity routine but present different conceptual messages for each day of the week. Simply play the appropriate video and have your students perform the routine for that day. The DVD also provides an instructional video for each week's routine. If your school has a physical education teacher, he or she may have taught the routine to students during the week before Wellness Week, in which case you won't have to use the instructional video. Otherwise, you can use it to help your students learn the routine.

In the instructional video, the instructor faces away from your students for some of the left–right movements. Explain to students that they should do those movements the same way the instructor does them. That is, when the instructor moves to the right, they should also move to the right. However, in the daily activity videos, the leaders face forward, so their left–right movements are in reverse (mirror image). While following along with the daily activity videos, your students should move in the opposite direction of the leaders for left–right movements. Keep in mind that although moving in the correct direction is desirable, the key is to get all kids moving regardless of the direction. If your students have a hard time performing the activity, feel free to replay the instructional video.

# Day **1** Lesson Plan

## OVERVIEW

* **Morning Activity Break**: La Raspa (DVD routine)
* **Afternoon Activity Break:** Itsy Bitsy Spider

## OBJECTIVES

Students will

* participate in 10 minutes of moderate to vigorous physical activity;
* repeat the message that being active keeps them alert and helps their hearts get strong;
* list two jobs in which workers are physically active; and
* participate in physical activity, making only supportive comments to themselves and others.

## RESOURCES

### Signs

 **General**

G2: Wellness Week

G3: Physical Activity Pyramid for Kids

G8: Healthy mind, healthy body, healthy heart . . . let's start!

 **Wellness Week 2 → Signs**

2.1: Physical Activity Pyramid: Make some activity vigorous!

2.2: Get your body moving!

* 2.3: Being active is a great start! Being active builds my heart!

* 2.4: If it makes you breathe hard and sweat, it helps your brain and body, you bet!

---

* Indicates signs used for chants

### Worksheets

The DVD includes black-and-white versions of today's signs that you can print and use as coloring worksheets. In addition, the DVD includes black-and-white versions of MyPyramid for Kids and the Physical Activity Pyramid for Kids for coloring.

 **Wellness Week 2 → Worksheets**

**teacher tip** • • •
Your enthusiasm will go a long way to "sell" physical activity as an important part of daily life. Focus on enjoying this active time yourself as well as on the importance of it for your students' minds and bodies! Emphasize this week's theme of vigorous activity—such as vigorous aerobics, sports, and recreation.

# MORNING ACTIVITY BREAK

**DVD Routine**: La Raspa

## Introduction

"This Wellness Week we're going to talk about movement that makes our hearts beat faster. We have a new video routine. Remember last time how it was a little hard at first, but as we practiced it every day, it got easier? That will happen this time as well. The more we practice, the easier it will be."

## Video Routine

The DVD has five versions of the La Raspa routine, one for each day of the week. It also has a special instructional version that teaches students how to do the routine.

1. Play the instructional routine. If the PE teacher has already taught the routine to the students, you can skip this step.
2. Play the Day 1 routine.

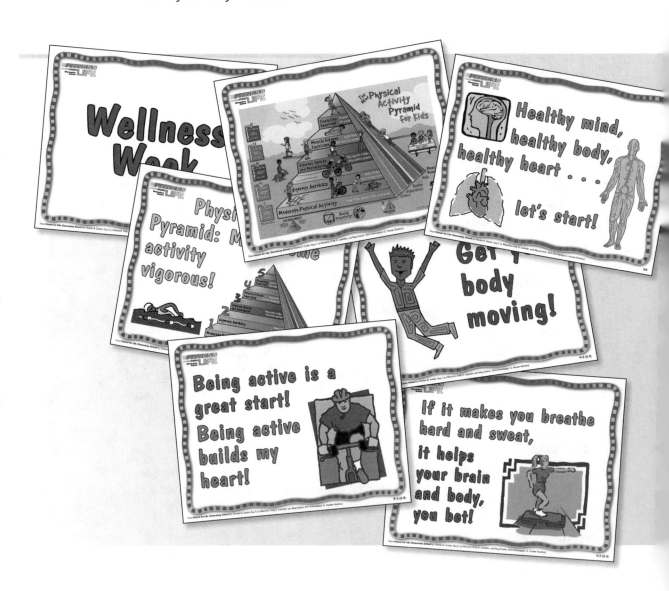

Each day the current version of the routine promotes a new and different message. Variations on the message play before the first routine, between routines, and after the last routine. For La Raspa, the Day 1 message is "Get your body moving," and the three variations are as follows:

* Whether you live in the city or on a farm, moving your body is a lucky charm.
* All little kids love to move around: rolling, running, jumping, and making fun sounds.
* When you're very active, you feel alert and alive; if it makes your heart beat faster, give a high five! If it makes you breathe hard and sweat, it helps your brain and body work well—you bet.

## Breathing

After finishing the routine, lead the class in breathing.

"Breathing deeply is important for our bodies, so we'll end every activity with a couple of deep breaths. Let's all breathe in deeply (count 1, 2), hold (count 1, 2), breathe out (count 1, 2), and hold (count 1, 2)." Repeat three times.

## Background Information

* U.S. Department of Health and Human Services guidelines (2008) recommend that children and adolescents should be involved in vigorous physical activity at least three days per week.
* According to the national guidelines, being physically active results in positive health benefits for children.
* Children tend to be active intermittently, especially during play. Play allows them to do a variety of activities that develop skills. It also allows them to be involved with brief periods of moderate to vigorous physical activity and rest that enables them to reach the guidelines.

## Discussion

* Point to the Physical Activity Pyramid for Kids. Show vigorous activity on steps 2 and 3, and emphasize that kids need some vigorous activity each day.
* "Can you feel your heart beating? Put your hand on your chest like this. Use your other hand to show me how fast it is beating like this." (Open and close your hand in time to your heart beat).
* "Why does your heart have to beat faster when you move around fast?"

## Chant

Chanting is a great way to reinforce messages. If you've posted the corresponding sign, point to it, and tell the students that when you say the first phrase, they should respond by saying the second phrase. Make it fun!

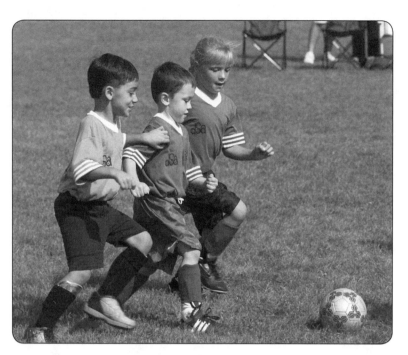

Get your body moving! Physical activity is beneficial to the body and the mind.

Teacher: "Being active is a great start!"

Students: "Being active builds my heart!"

Teacher: "If it makes you breathe hard and sweat . . ."

Students: ". . . it helps your brain and body—you bet!"

Practice several times until the students respond easily to your prompt.

## Closure

Closure provides an opportunity to focus one more time on the main message of the lesson by using compliments, reviewing messages, and making suggestions for doing activity at home. Closure also includes a brief preview of what's coming in the next lesson to help students see connections and begin to prepare for future lessons.

### Compliments

"You did a great job following the video and got some vigorous exercise. You were working hard. I could tell by how fast your hearts were beating. That will make your hearts even stronger."

### Take It Home

"Since we all need to get some vigorous physical activity, let's think of things you can do at home that will make your heart beat faster."

> ⟳ **review** • • •
> "Today we talked about activities that make your heart beat faster. Did you feel your heart beating fast? What else did you feel?"

### Preview

"Tomorrow we're going to do the La Raspa routine again. We'll get better and better."

## AFTERNOON ACTIVITY BREAK

**Activity**: Itsy Bitsy Spider

Perform in the afternoon or at some other time during the day when the students need a physical activity break.

Use large motions rather than finger motions so that the children get more physical activity. Teach children the song and motions to Itsy Bitsy Spider.

* "The itsy, bitsy spider climbed up the water spout." (Pretend to be climbing: reach up and pull down with hands, and lift knees high as if climbing.)
* "Down came the rain and washed the spider out." (Bring hands from above the head to near the knees.)

* "Out came the sun and dried up all the rain." (Make a big sun with hands.)
* "And the itsy, bitsy spider climbed up the spout again." (Climb up again.)
* Repeat several times.

**observation • • •**

We're talking about vigorous activity this week. Look around to determine if the children are working at more than a walk level. If so, reinforce how great it is for your body to do vigorous exercise. If not encourage them to lift their knees higher, move a little faster, use their arms, and so on to increase their activity.

## Breathing

After finishing the activity, lead the class in breathing.

"Breathing deeply is important for our bodies, so we'll end every activity with a couple of deep breaths. Let's all breathe in deeply (count 1, 2), hold (count 1, 2), breathe out (count 1, 2), and hold (count 1, 2)." Repeat three times.

## Closure

"Thanks for working so hard and showing such good body control. You all did that without any problems even though we are in a small space. Nice work. I wonder what it would be like to be a spider on a spider web. Let's look for spider webs on the playground, and if we find one, carefully watch what the spiders do."

# ADDITIONAL ACTIVITIES

See appendix A for additional enriching and integrative outdoor activities. For more information, go to www.fitnessforlife.org.

# 2 WELLNESS WEEK

## Day 2 Lesson Plan

WEEK 2 · DAY 2

### OVERVIEW

* **Morning Activity Break**: La Raspa (DVD routine)
* **Afternoon Activity Break**: Pattern Practice

### OBJECTIVES

Students will

* participate in 10 minutes of moderate to vigorous physical activity;
* repeat the message that practicing helps them get better;
* identify one way to tell if they are exercising vigorously (heart beating faster, sweating);
* participate in physical activity, making only supportive comments to themselves and others;
* identify the next movement in a repeating ABC pattern and move correctly to the ABC pattern; and
* make a reasonable estimate of the number of marching steps taken in 10 seconds and check the estimate by counting steps.

### RESOURCES

#### Signs

 **Wellness Week 2 → Signs**

* 2.5: The more you practice, the better you play; practice, practice every day!

---

* Indicates sign used for chant

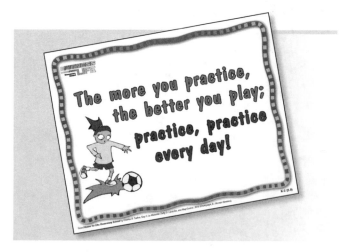

#### Worksheets

The DVD includes a black-and-white version of today's sign that you can print and use as a coloring worksheet. In addition, the DVD includes black-and-white versions of MyPyramid for Kids and the Physical Activity Pyramid for Kids for coloring.

 **Wellness Week 2 → Worksheets**

60

# MORNING ACTIVITY BREAK

**DVD Routine**: La Raspa

## Introduction

"Yesterday we talked about moving enough to have our hearts start beating faster. Doing activities where our hearts beat more quickly makes our hearts stronger. And the more we practice, the better we get. Can you think of something that you didn't know how to do and then after you practiced it, you were able to do it?"

Solicit answers.

"Today we're doing the La Raspa routine again. Since we already did it once it will be a little easier to do today. We're getting better at it because we are practicing it every day. Yesterday you all showed me good body control. You were in control of your body and didn't bump anyone else. That's great! It kept everyone safe."

## Video Routine

The DVD has five versions of the La Raspa routine, one for each day of the week. It also has a special instructional version that teaches students how to do the routine.

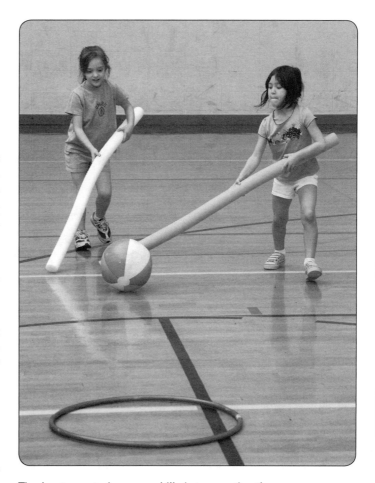

The best way to improve skills is to practice them.

1. If the students have not done this week's routine before, play the instructional routine. If the PE teacher has already taught the routine to the students, or if they have already practiced the instructional routine with you, you can skip this step.

2. Play the Day 2 routine.

Each day the current version of the routine promotes a new and different message. Variations on the message play before the first routine, between routines, and after the last routine. For La Raspa, the Day 2 message is "Get better with practice," and the three variations are as follows:

✳ Do it once, then do it twice; practice, practice is good advice.

✳ The more you practice, the better you play; practice, practice every day.

✳ Practice means trying again and again until you are good. Try it, try it—I knew you could.

## Breathing

After finishing the routine, lead the class in breathing.

"Breathing deeply is important for our bodies, so we'll end every activity with a couple of deep breaths. Let's all breathe in deeply (count 1, 2), hold (count 1, 2), breathe out (count 1, 2), and hold (count 1, 2)." Repeat three times.

WEEK **2** • DAY **2**

## Background Information

❋ When learning a new skill, spacing out practice with rest is more effective than trying to practice without any rest.

❋ When learning a new skill, the learner tends to think a lot about how to do the skill which can negatively impact performance; as the individual continues to practice, the skill becomes more automatic and requires less thought.

❋ Setting specific goals can motivate an individual to practice a skill.

## Discussion

❋ "Put your hand on your heart. With your other hand, show me how fast your heart is beating."

❋ "What other activities do you do that make your heart beat faster?"

❋ "Did you ever make a mistake when you were doing something new? Did you ever practice something that you weren't very good at and then get better at it?" (Talk about learning to write or count or ride a bike.)

## Chant

Chanting is a great way to reinforce messages. If you've posted the corresponding sign, point to it, and tell the students that when you say the first phrase, they should respond by saying the second phrase. Make it fun!

> **teacher tip · · ·**
> Chants can be fun and really help remind us of important points. Be enthusiastic, use different accents, and allow the students to shout back their response sometimes. Encourage students to teach the chants to their families.

Teacher: "The more you practice, the better you play."

Students: "Practice, practice every day!"

Practice several times until the students respond easily to your prompt.

## Closure

Closure provides an opportunity to focus one more time on the main message of the lesson by using compliments, reviewing messages, and making suggestions for doing activity at home. Closure also includes a brief preview of what's coming in the next lesson to help students see connections and begin to prepare for future lessons.

### *Compliments*

"You did a great job following the video. Practice helps us get better at things. By Friday, we'll be really good at this routine because we'll practice it every day this week."

> **review · · ·**
> "Today we got our hearts beating fast and talked about how practice helps us get better at doing things. When your heart beats fast, you usually breathe faster, too. Can you feel your breathing slowing down now that you are not active?"

### *Take It Home*

"Think about something you'd like to get better at. Could you practice it at home today?"

### *Preview*

"Tomorrow we will practice La Raspa again."

# AFTERNOON ACTIVITY BREAK

**Activity**: Pattern Practice

Perform in the afternoon or at some other time during the day when the students need a physical activity break.

"Do you remember the movement patterns we did last Wellness Week? Remember, we had a letter pattern: A, B, A, B, A, B, A, __; what do you think is next? Yes, B. OK!

> **⊗ interdisciplinary** • • •
> This activity helps students practice patterns in movement. Being able to recognize, follow, and create patterns are also important skills in math.

Let's do our AB pattern with movements, using good body control. A is stand up, and B is sit down. Stand up, sit down, stand up, sit down, stand up, sit down, stand up, _____; what's next? Right, sit down. Let's do another pattern. Jump and put your feet apart, now feet together, now feet apart, together, apart, together, apart, ____; what's next? Right, together. Let's do it 10 times.

Let's do an ABC pattern this time. Let's make A stepping on your left foot, B stepping on your right foot, and C giving a little jump. Let's try it. Step on your left foot, then step on your right foot, then give a little jump. Left, right, jump, left, right, __; what's next? Correct; jump. Now you help me make up an ABC pattern. What will our A movement be? Our B movement? What will our C movement be? ABC ABC A__; What's next? Yes, B, and then C. Patterns can be hard to do at first, but if we keep practicing them, we get better at them, and they seem easier."

Write the pattern on the board. Talk about patterns, how to extend them, and how you can look at them in different ways such as single units, or as groups of units as in A B C A B C = ABC ABC.

## Breathing

After finishing the activity, lead the class in breathing.

"Breathing deeply is important for our bodies, so we'll end every activity with a couple of deep breaths. Let's all breathe in deeply

> **👁 observation** • • •
> We're talking about vigorous activity this week. Look around to see if the children are working above the level of a walk. If so, reinforce how great it is to do vigorous exercise. If not, choose more vigorous movements. Encourage them to lift their knees higher, move a little faster, use their arms, and so on to increase their activity.

(count 1, 2), hold (count 1, 2), breathe out (count 1, 2), and hold (count 1, 2)." Repeat three times.

## Closure

"Thanks for showing such good body control. You all did that without any problems even though we are in a small space. You paid careful attention to the pattern and used your thinking skills to figure out what the next part of the pattern was. Since you have such good body control and pay attention to the patterns, we can keep doing active games in the classroom. I won't have to worry about you getting hurt when you are moving in this little space."

# ADDITIONAL ACTIVITIES

See appendix A for additional enriching and integrative outdoor activities. For more information, go to www.fitnessforlife.org.

WEEK **2** • DAY **2**

# 2 WELLNESS WEEK

## Day 3 Lesson Plan

### OVERVIEW

* **Morning Activity Break**: La Raspa (DVD routine)
* **Eat Well Wednesday Class Discussion**: Whole Grains and Breakfast
* **Eat Well Wednesday Activity**: Healthy Breakfast Promotion
* **Afternoon Activity Break**: Simon Says

### OBJECTIVES

Students will

* participate in 10 minutes of moderate to vigorous physical activity;
* repeat (correctly) the message that their bodies need some good fat, but some kinds of fat are bad, and they shouldn't eat them very often (the bad kinds of fat are trans fat, saturated fat, and animal fat);
* name three foods that are good to eat every day;
* practice decision making and attention by responding with movement on appropriate verbal cues (Simon Says) and not responding when the cue is missing;
* identify the color of the grain stripe on MyPyramid (orange);
* identify the color of the oils stripe on MyPyramid (yellow); and
* understand that the body uses grains for energy.

### RESOURCES

#### Signs

 **General**

G4: MyPyramid for Kids

G5: Eat Well Wednesday

G10: ABCs of Nutrition

 **Wellness Week 2 → Signs**

2.6: Orange is for grains!

2.7: Make half your grains whole!

2.8: Avoid empty calories!

\* 2.9: Some fats are good, some fats are bad. What kind of fats has your body had?

2.10: Break the fast with breakfast!

---

\* Indicates sign used for chant

## Worksheets

The DVD includes black-and-white versions of today's signs that you can print and use as coloring worksheets. In addition, the DVD includes black-and-white versions of MyPyramid for Kids and the Physical Activity Pyramid for Kids for coloring.

 **Wellness Week 2 → Worksheets**

# MORNING ACTIVITY BREAK

**DVD Routine**: La Raspa

## Introduction

"Wellness Week reminds us of things we should be doing every week and every day. Yesterday, we talked about how important practice is when we are learning new things. We've also talked about the importance of eating fruits and vegetables. Today we'll talk about another part of food called fat. Some fat is important to our body, but some kinds cause problems. Doing the routine should be easier today because this is our third day trying it. Show me your good body control again today."

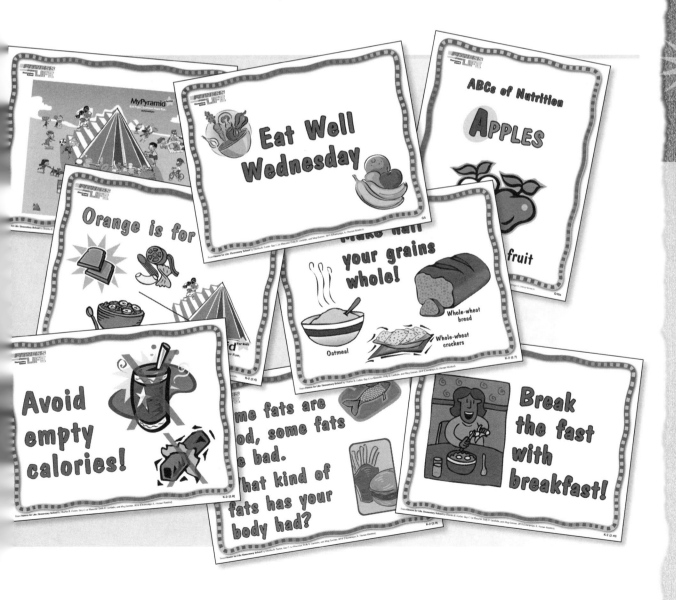

## Video Routine

The DVD has five versions of the La Raspa routine, one for each day of the week. It also has a special instructional version that teaches students how to do the routine.

1. If the students have not done this week's routine before, play the instructional routine. If the PE teacher has already taught the routine to the students, or if they have already practiced the instructional routine with you, you can skip this step.
2. Play the Day 3 routine.

Each day the current version of the routine promotes a new and different message. Variations on the message play before the first routine, between routines, and after the last routine. For La Raspa, the Day 3 message is "Foods with fats" (discussions also feature grains), and the three variations are as follows:

＊ Some foods with fats are good; some fats are bad. What kind of fats has your body had?

＊ Some foods with fats are good; some fats are bad. What kind of fats has your body had?

＊ Your body needs fat for energy, protection, and warmth. Fats are found in many foods like muffins, bacon, cheese, and ice cream. Eating too much fatty food is not good for your body.

**observation** • • •

Look around the room. Are the children showing good body control? Are there any parts of the routine that are particularly hard, creating stumbling blocks for the students? Note any so you can either have the students practice that piece or modify the routine to allow them to flow through it.

## Breathing

After finishing the routine, lead the class in breathing.

"Breathing deeply is important for our bodies, so we'll end every activity with a couple of deep breaths. Let's all breathe in deeply (count 1, 2), hold (count 1, 2), breathe out (count 1, 2), and hold (count 1, 2)." Repeat three times.

## Background Information

＊ Oils are represented by the narrow yellow color band in MyPyramid. Oils are not a food group but are pictured to make people aware of oils in foods and the need to limit them in food.

＊ Fat contains a lot of calories in a small package. (There are nine calories in a gram of fat compared to four calories in a gram of protein and carbohydrate.)

＊ Trans fats and saturated fats are bad kinds of fat.

＊ Your body stores energy in the form of fat.

＊ There is healthy fat (omega-3) that helps reduce the risk of heart disease.

## Discussion

＊ "There is good fat in fish and olive oil. Can you remember any names of fish that people eat? Raise your hand if you have heard of salmon, trout, red fish, or flounder."

＊ "Hamburgers, french fries, and ice cream have some of the problem fat in them, so it's important not to eat too much of those foods."

## Chant

Chanting is a great way to reinforce messages. If you've posted the corresponding sign, point to it, and tell the students that when you say the first phrase, they should respond by saying the second phrase. Make it fun!

Teacher: "Some fats are good, some fats are bad."

Students: "What kind of fats has your body had?"

Practice several times until the students respond easily to your prompt.

> **observation** • • •
> We're talking about vigorous activity this week. Look around to see if the children are working above the level of a walk. If so, reinforce how great it is to do vigorous exercise. If not, encourage them to lift their knees higher, move a little faster, use their arms, and so on to increase their activity.

## Closure

Closure provides an opportunity to focus one more time on the main message of the lesson by using compliments, reviewing messages, and making suggestions for doing activity at home. Closure also includes a brief preview of what's coming in the next lesson to help students see connections and begin to prepare for future lessons.

### *Compliments*

"You did lots of good exercising while doing La Raspa."

### *Take It Home*

"Remember it's great to be active at home and to invite others to be active with you. It is also good to eat healthy foods. Maybe you can have some baked fries instead of fried french fries next time. Talk to your family about it."

### *Preview*

"Tomorrow we're going to be talking about the importance of exercising your heart."

# EAT WELL WEDNESDAY

Each Wednesday all teachers and staff are encouraged to emphasize the weekly nutrition message. Special schoolwide events (e.g., a lunch salad bar or healthy snack preparation) may be planned by the wellness coordinator. Teachers are encouraged to support these Eat Well Wednesday events and plan special Eat Well Wednesday events in their classrooms, emphasizing sound nutrition.

## Eat Well Wednesday Class Discussion

**Nutrition Topic:** Whole Grains and Breakfast

### *Introduction*

Introduce MyPyramid and the healthy food group of the week—grains. MyPyramid is a nutrition guideline used to promote healthy eating and to introduce the five food groups (plus oils): grains, vegetables, fruits, milk, and meat and beans. Each food group represents a different nutritional category. Discuss the importance of grains in the diet. Also discuss the importance of a healthy breakfast to start the day.

### *Background Information*

* When you treat your body well, it will grow, keep itself strong, and heal itself when it gets hurt.
* Nutrients are elements in healthy foods with special jobs. There are six nutrient types (carbohydrate, vitamins, minerals, fat, protein, and water).

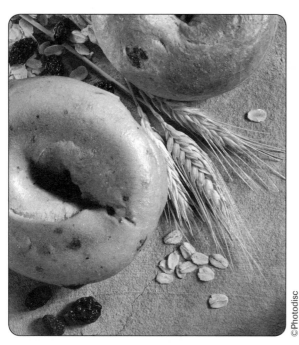

Grains are an important source of carbohydrate, the body's main source of energy.

©Photodisc

✳ By eating a wide variety of foods, every color every day, your body receives all the nutrients it needs to learn, move, and grow.

✳ Grains are important to your body. Your body uses calories, the energy found in food. The body's main source of energy is from the starches in carbohydrate, found in grains and vegetables.

✳ Grains are foods like cereal, bread, and pasta.

✳ Processed grains have some of the nutrients stripped out of them. Whole grains have all the parts of the grain and lots more nutrients for your body. At least half of the grains you eat each day should be whole grains.

✳ Grains are a major component of the diet and are represented by the wide orange color band on MyPyramid.

✳ Breakfast is the most important meal of the day, yet many children and adults extend the "fast" that started while they were sleeping and start their day on an empty stomach.

✳ Breakfast gets you ready to learn, move, and grow.

✳ For breakfast, always include whole grains, fiber, and protein. Have a bowl of whole-wheat cereal with low-fat milk and bananas, a slice of whole-wheat toast with melted cheese and apple slices, brown rice and beans with fruit, yogurt topped with a favorite whole-wheat cereal, or a whole-wheat pita stuffed with scrambled eggs.

### Discussion

✳ "Why do you think breakfast is the most important meal of the day?"

✳ "What are some of the foods from the different parts of the food pyramid that we might have at breakfast?"

✳ "Turn to your neighbors and tell them what you had for breakfast. How healthy was it? If it wasn't too healthy, how would you change it to make it healthy?"

✳ "Turn to your neighbor and name three whole grains." (e.g., brown rice, oatmeal, popcorn, whole wheat bread, pasta or crackers, barley)

✳ "Do you eat whole grains at home? Can you give some examples?" (Answers might include whole-grain cereal, whole-grain tortillas, or whole-grain bread.)

✳ "Did you eat any whole grains yesterday?"

### Take It Home

✳ "Find out from your family members their favorite whole-grain cereals."

✳ "Go shopping with your family and buy one new whole-grain item."

**↻ review • • •**
"Grains are good for you; they have a wide band in MyPyramid because they should be a big part of your diet. Whole grains are especially good for you. Exercising and eating lots of fruits and veggies and not too much fat like that found in meat, cheese, and pastry is important every day. Avoid foods that have a lot of fat." (Examples of high-fat foods include butter and meat with fat.)

### Eat Well Wednesday Schoolwide Activity

During Wellness Week 2, healthy breakfasts will be featured in the cafeteria.

# AFTERNOON ACTIVITY BREAK

**Activity**: Simon Says

Perform in the afternoon or at some other time during the day when the students need a physical activity break.

Begin by explaining how the game works. Tell them that when you start an instruction with "Simon says," they should do what you say. But if you simply tell them to do something, such as "Wave your arms," they shouldn't respond. Then lead them through several examples so they understand how the game works. For instance, if you say, "Simon says, 'Put your hands on your hips,'" the students should put their hands on their hips. But if you say, "Put your hands on your hips," the students should not do it.

If students make mistakes, just say "Oops," laugh with them, and then go on with the next action. Include lots of jumping up and down and marching activities since this week we are talking about vigorous physical activity. (Some activities you might consider: march, jump five times, run in place, reach high, jump with feet apart, jump with feet together, touch head, shoulders, knees, or toes. Ask them to "feel your heart, and if you can feel it beat, show me its beat by opening and closing your other hand whenever it beats.") End up with more gentle movements so they calm down slowly, and the heart slows down.

If students have the basic idea, use shapes or other items instead of saying "Simon says." Have students do the movement when you hold up any shape except a square, and have them do as many repetitions of the movement as there are points on the shape. For example, when you hold up an octagon and say "Do jumping jacks," students would do eight jumping jacks. But if you hold up a square, they should not do any jumping jacks.

> **⊠ interdisciplinary • • •**
> This activity includes movement and helps students practice categorizing skills since they have to put the instructions into one of two categories: instructions to follow and instructions to ignore. The activity also provides practice in number operations by using various methods for defining the number of times to do each movement.

## Breathing

After finishing the activity, lead the class in breathing.

"Breathing deeply is important for our bodies, so we'll end every activity with a couple of deep breaths. Let's all breathe in deeply (count 1, 2), hold (count 1, 2), breathe out (count 1, 2), and hold (count 1, 2)." Repeat three times.

## Closure

"Thanks for showing such good body control. You paid careful attention to what Simon said to do. That's careful listening. Careful listening helps you learn lots of new things. You also helped your heart get stronger by having it work hard."

> **⑦ comprehension check • • •**
> "Show me what you will do if I say, 'Simon says, "Touch your shoulders."' Show me what you will do if I say, 'Touch your knees' without saying, 'Simon says.'"

# ADDITIONAL ACTIVITIES

See appendix A for additional enriching and integrative outdoor activities. For more information, go to www.fitnessforlife.org.

WEEK 2 • DAY 3

# 2 WELLNESS WEEK

## Day 4 Lesson Plan

### OVERVIEW

* **Morning Activity Break**: La Raspa (DVD routine)
* **Afternoon Activity Break**: Follow the Leader

### OBJECTIVES

Students will

* participate in 10 minutes of moderate to vigorous physical activity;
* repeat the message that exercising their hearts helps make their hearts strong;
* name two activities in which their hearts are getting good exercise;
* participate in physical activity, making only supportive comments to themselves and others; and
* describe the importance of having a standard unit of measure.

### RESOURCES

**Signs**

 **Wellness Week 2 → Signs**

2.11: Making your heart beat fast helps your body last!

2.12: A healthy heart is a happy heart!

* 2.13: Exercising your heart daily really pays. Your heart will thank you in many ways!

* Indicates sign used for chant

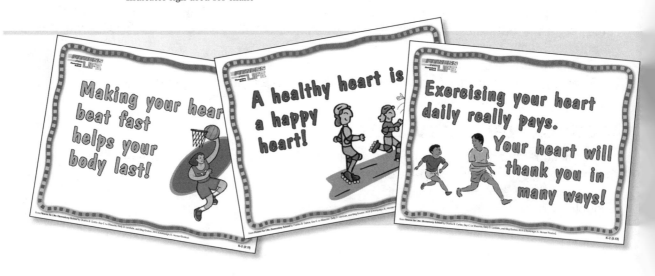

70

## Worksheets

The DVD includes black-and-white versions of today's signs that you can print and use as coloring worksheets. In addition, the DVD includes black-and-white versions of MyPyramid for Kids and the Physical Activity Pyramid for Kids for coloring.

 **Wellness Week 2 → Worksheets**

# MORNING ACTIVITY BREAK

**DVD Routine**: La Raspa

## Introduction

"Yesterday we talked about what kinds of fat are in foods. Some fat is important for our bodies, but some kinds are harmful. They make blocks in the tubes that take the blood from our hearts around our bodies. Exercising our hearts by being very active helps keep our blood vessels clean so the blood can go where it needs to. When we do La Raspa today, enjoy your heart pumping fast. It's good for your heart to beat fast when you are active."

## Video Routine

The DVD has five versions of the La Raspa routine, one for each day of the week. It also has a special instructional version that teaches students how to do the routine.

1. If the students have not done this week's routine before, play the instructional routine. If the PE teacher has already taught the routine to the students, or if they have already practiced the instructional routine with you, you can skip this step.
2. Play the Day 4 routine.

Each day the current version of the routine promotes a new and different message. Variations on the message play before the first routine, between routines, and after the last routine. For La Raspa, the Day 4 message is "Exercise your heart," and the three variations are as follows:

* Exercising your heart really pays—your heart will thank you in so many ways!

* Moving your body gets your heart thump, thump, thumping. Your cardio pump just keeps on pumping!

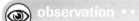 **observation** • • •
Look around the room. Are the students doing the activity with ease? Tell them how well they are doing and how much better they have gotten with practice.

* Playing hard and being active are a good start; it gets your blood pumping and builds a strong heart. Making your heart beat fast helps your body last.

## Breathing

After finishing the routine, lead the class in breathing.

"Breathing deeply is important for our bodies, so we'll end every activity with a couple of deep breaths. Let's all breathe in deeply (count 1, 2), hold (count 1, 2), breathe out (count 1, 2), and hold (count 1, 2)." Repeat three times.

WEEK **2** • DAY **4**

## Background Information

✳ Regular exercise strengthens the heart. When the heart is stronger, it can pump more blood with each beat. So if it is stronger, your resting heart rate is lower.

✳ Resting heart rates are usually between 60 and 80 beats per minute. Everyone is different, but if you are fit, your heart rate will be lower than if you are not.

✳ With a stronger heart, you can play and be active longer without getting tired.

## Discussion

✳ "Did your heart beat fast during the routine?"

✳ "What other activities make your heart beat fast?"

✳ "What are your favorite activities that make your heart beat fast?"

✳ "Did you eat a healthy breakfast this morning? What did you have?"

✳ "What fruits and veggies have you been eating?"

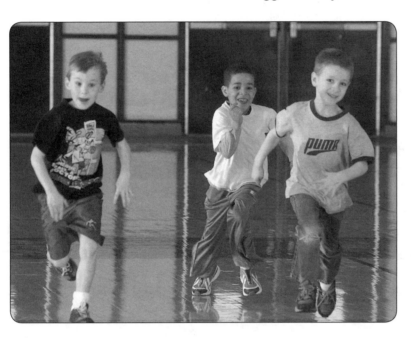

Vigorous aerobic exercise will improve heart health.

## Chant

Chanting is a great way to reinforce messages. If you've posted the corresponding sign, point to it, and tell the students that when you say the first phrase, they should respond by saying the second phrase. Make it fun!

Teacher: "Exercising your heart daily really pays."

Students: "Your heart will thank you in many ways!"

Practice several times until the students respond easily to your prompt.

## Closure

Closure provides an opportunity to focus one more time on the main message of the lesson by using compliments, reviewing messages, and making suggestions for doing activity at home. Closure also includes a brief preview of what's coming in the next lesson to help students see connections and begin to prepare for future lessons.

**review** • • •
"Being active so your heart beats faster and eating healthy foods are good things to do. How do you think being fit feels? Do you feel it in your legs? In your head?"

### Compliments

"You're getting so good at the routine that it looks like you can almost do it without thinking about it. You are getting good enough to sing or hum along as you are doing it. It's hard to do that when you are first learning the routine. Your practice has helped you learn the routine so you don't have to concentrate on it so much anymore."

### Take It Home

"Help people at your house remember to be active and eat healthy every day."

### Preview

"This afternoon we'll play Follow the Leader and tomorrow we'll do La Raspa."

> **⭐ teacher tip • • •**
>
> Sharing positive expectations and describing helpful behavior, how it looks and sounds, can go a long way to helping children enjoy participation in movement settings. For example, you might say something like: "Sometimes things are hard to do. What could a person do to get back on track after she made a mistake? What might you say to someone to encourage him to keep trying when he was getting tired?"

## AFTERNOON ACTIVITY BREAK

**Activity**: Follow the Leader

Perform in the afternoon or at some other time during the day when the students need a physical activity break.

Tell the students that in Follow the Leader, they should do exactly what you do. Then start the activity. "Ready? Here we go!"

Start with simple actions. Try to do at least eight counts of each movement. For example: put your hands in the air and wave them back and forth 1, 2, 3, 4, 5, 6, 7, 8; march in place 1, 2, 3, 4, 5, 6, 7, 8; clap your hands 1, 2, 3, 4, 5, 6, 7, 8; run in place; count forward and backward. Talk about counting different ways. Since we are talking about vigorous exercise this week, include lots of running in place and jumping. When you get near the end of the exercise, do slower movements to allow their hearts to slow down again. Tell them you are doing this.

### Breathing

After finishing the activity, lead the class in breathing.

"Breathing deeply is important for our bodies, so we'll end every activity with a couple of deep breaths. Let's all breathe in deeply (count 1, 2), hold (count 1, 2), breathe out (count 1, 2), and hold (count 1, 2)." Repeat three times.

### Closure

"You worked hard today and made your heart beat fast. Yesterday you paid careful attention to what Simon said. Today you worked hard and paid careful attention to what I was doing. That's careful watching. Careful watching helps you learn lots of new things."

> **👁 observation • • •**
>
> We're talking about vigorous activity this week. Look around to see if the children are working above the level of a walk. If so, reinforce how great it is to do vigorous exercise. If not, encourage them to lift knees their higher, move a little faster, use their arms, and so on to increase their activity.

## ADDITIONAL ACTIVITIES

See appendix A for additional enriching and integrative outdoor activities. For more information, go to www.fitnessforlife.org.

# ☀ WELLNESS WEEK

## Day 5 Lesson Plan ● ● ● ● ● ● ● ● ● ● ● ● ● ● ●

## OVERVIEW

* ✳ **Get Fit Friday Activity**: TEAM Time 2: Big Kids Lead
* ✳ **Morning Activity Break**: La Raspa (DVD routine)
* ✳ **Afternoon Activity Break**: Shirt Color Lineup

## OBJECTIVES

Students will

* ✳ participate in 10 minutes of moderate to vigorous physical activity;
* ✳ move fluidly and confidently during the video routine;
* ✳ repeat the message that the secret to success is trying;
* ✳ demonstrate understanding of a bar graph by identifying the most common shirt color;
* ✳ participate in physical activity, making only supportive comments to themselves and others; and
* ✳ be members of the team who try to help the team accomplish the task (Shirt Color Lineup).

## RESOURCES

### Signs

 **General**

G6: TEAM Time: Together Everyone Achieves More
G7: Get Fit Friday

 **Wellness Week 2 → Signs**

\* 2.14: Keep on going to get fit. Never give up! Never quit!

---

\* Indicates sign used for chant

### Worksheets

The DVD includes a black-and-white version of today's sign that you can print and use as a coloring worksheet. In addition, the DVD includes black-and-white versions of MyPyramid for Kids and the Physical Activity Pyramid for Kids for coloring.

 **Wellness Week 2 → Worksheets**

# GET FIT FRIDAY

During each Wellness Week, Day 5 (typically Friday) is known as Get Fit Friday. On this day, a schoolwide event focusing on physical activity will be planned by the wellness coordinator. The Get Fit Friday activities are called TEAM Time activities (TEAM stands for Together Everyone Achieves More).

During Wellness Week 2, the TEAM Time activity planned for Get Fit Friday is called Big Kids Lead. The wellness coordinator will lead the activity at the beginning of the school day with the help of students in fifth and sixth grades. All students in the school will congregate outside or in the gym or multipurpose room so that they all can participate together. The TEAM Time activity includes a warm-up, a special routine called Colors, and a cool-down.

In addition to supporting Big Kids Lead, mention the TEAM Time activity as you discuss the video routine messages during the morning activity break.

# MORNING ACTIVITY BREAK

**DVD Routine**: La Raspa

## Introduction

"We've been doing the La Raspa video all week, so today we should be getting pretty good at it. I hope you can sing or hum along as you do it. Try it. Trying hard means paying attention to what we are doing, but when we have done that a lot and we get really good, sometimes we just do it without even having to think about it. Let's see if we can do this routine easily."

## Video Routine

The DVD has five versions of the La Raspa routine, one for each day of the week. It also has a special instructional version that teaches students how to do the routine.

1. If the students have not done this week's routine before, play the instructional routine. If the PE teacher has already taught the routine to the students, or if they have already practiced the instructional routine with you, you can skip this step.

2. Play the Day 5 routine.

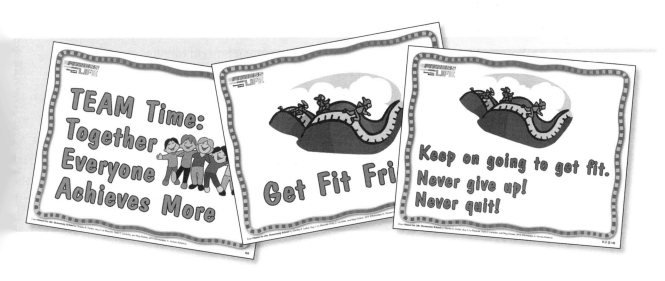

WEEK **2** • DAY **5**

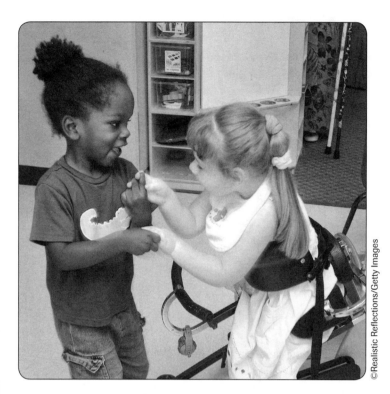

Never, ever give up! Trying hard will make you proud.

Each day the current version of the routine promotes a new and different message. Variations on the message play before the first routine, between routines, and after the last routine. For La Raspa, the Day 5 message is "Never, ever give up," and the three variations are as follows:

❋ Never give up, say it out loud; trying hard will make you proud.

❋ Do your best, try hard, never quit; being active will get you fit.

❋ That means keep going even if it's hard, whether it's inside or in the yard. Keep on going to get fit—never give up, never quit.

## Breathing

After finishing the routine, lead the class in breathing.

"Breathing deeply is important for our bodies, so we'll end every activity with a couple of deep breaths. Let's all breathe in deeply (count 1, 2), hold (count 1, 2), breathe out (count 1, 2), and hold (count 1, 2)." Repeat three times.

## Background Information

❋ You never know what you can do unless you keep trying.

❋ Keep going and trying, that's how you get better!

❋ Sometimes when you try something new, it's hard. But if you keep trying, it becomes easier to do!

❋ Your muscles have memories, and if you do something over and over, your muscles and your brain help remember how to do it.

## Discussion

❋ "Our class is a team. What are some things we can do to help each other keep trying?"

❋ "Has anyone ever said something that helped you keep trying at something that was hard?"

## Chant

Chanting is a great way to reinforce messages. Use your favorite chants from previous lessons. If you've posted the corresponding sign, point to it, and tell the students that when you say the first phrase, they should respond by saying the second phrase. Make it fun!

Teacher: "Being active is a great start!"

Students: "Being active builds my heart!"

Teacher: "Some fats are good, some fats are bad."

Students: "What kind of fats has your body had?"

Teacher: "Exercising your heart daily really pays."

Students: "Your heart will thank you in many ways!"

Teacher: "Keep on going to get fit."

Students: "Never give up! Never quit!"

Practice several times until the students respond easily to your prompt.

## Closure

Closure provides an opportunity to focus one more time on the main message of the lesson by using compliments, reviewing messages, and making suggestions for doing activity at home. Closure also includes a brief

> **teacher tip • • •**
> "Nice time" refers to taking a few minutes to allow and encourage students to compliment each other on their work. Starting with a stem such as "I'd like to compliment _____ because she did a great job of _____" teaches the students how to identify a particular action to compliment. If you honor this time, the students will, too.

preview of what's coming in the next lesson to help students see connections and begin to prepare for future lessons.

### Compliments

"You're getting so good at the routine that you can almost do it without thinking about it. As a class, we are looking good!"

### Take It Home

* "Check to see what whole-grain foods you have at home."
* "Have you ever said 'no' to french fries or another food high in fat? If you answered, 'yes,' which ones did you turn down?"

> **review • • •**
> "Think about your body. What things do you feel when you have been very active? For instance, you might be hot and sweaty, or breathing hard. We've been talking about vigorous activity where you move around enough to get your heart beating faster, and you get at least a little sweaty. This week we did the La Raspa routine. We also talked about our bodies needing some good kinds of fat but that there is other fat that isn't very good for us."

* "Make a list of the activities that you do at home, such as taking a walk or playing with someone at home after school."

### Preview

"During the next Wellness Week, we'll talk about getting our muscles stronger."

## AFTERNOON ACTIVITY BREAK

**Activity**: Shirt Color Lineup

Perform in the afternoon or at some other time during the day when the students need a physical activity break.

"Remember last Wellness Week we lined up in alphabetical order. We're going to line up in a different way today. I'm going to tell you how to line up, and I want you to figure out where you should get in line. This time, let's line up by the colors of our shirts. Here's a rainbow." (Show a picture of a rainbow—Roy G. Biv is an easy way to remember the order of the colors: red, orange, yellow, green, blue, indigo, and violet.)

WEEK **2** • DAY **5**

(X) **interdisciplinary** • • •

This activity requires practice in sequencing as well as movement.

"When I say the color of your shirt, come get in line. If your shirt has more than one color, choose the color that seems the brightest or the one that is your favorite to decide when to line up. We'll start with reds right here, and make the line go that way. Ready, red—all the reds come line up. Next, orange, yellow, green, blue, indigo, and violet. Let's put black, gray, tan, and white at the end. Look at our rainbow!

"Now, let's clap once, jump two times, march three times, and run in place four times. Let's repeat that pattern. Clap once, jump two times, march three times, and run four times. If we were to add one more movement to our pattern like waving, how many times do you think we would do it? Right, five, because we did the first thing one time, the second thing two times, the third thing three times, and the fourth thing four times, so now we would do the fifth thing five times."

You can also use number operations when telling the students the number of times to do something (e.g., instead telling them four times, use two plus two). Have students use addition, subtraction, less than, more than, and so on to determine the number of times to do each exercise.

(◉) **observation** • • •

We're talking about vigorous activity this week. Look around to see if the children are working at more than a walk level. If so, reinforce how great it is to do vigorous exercise. If not, encourage them to lift their knees higher, move a little faster, use their arms, and so on to increase their activity.

## Breathing

After finishing the activity, lead the class in breathing.

"Breathing deeply is important for our bodies, so we'll end every activity with a couple of deep breaths. Let's all breathe in deeply (count 1, 2), hold (count 1, 2), breathe out (count 1, 2), and hold (count 1, 2)." Repeat three times.

## Closure

"You are good listeners and thinkers. Thanks for showing such good body control. On Wednesday, you listened carefully when we played Simon Says. Yesterday, you watched carefully when we played Follow the Leader. Today, you worked as a team, and we made a rainbow of our shirts. Working as a team means doing our part like going to the right place in the rainbow of shirts."

# ADDITIONAL ACTIVITIES

See appendix A for additional enriching and integrative outdoor activities. For more information, go to www.fitnessforlife.org.

# WELLNESS WEEK

## 3

## Fitness for Life Elementary School

## Week 3 Overview

Table 2.3 is a summary chart of the Wellness Week 3 activities for the second grade classroom. Pages 83 through 106 provide the daily lesson plans for each day of week 3.

- Week 3 physical activity theme: Muscle fitness and flexibility exercises
- Week 3 nutrition theme: Foods for strong bones and muscles

## Week 3 NASPE Standards

Week 3 activities meet the National Association for Sport and Physical Education (NASPE) standards listed here. For full standards and specific performance indicators (e.g., 1A through 6G), see appendix B.

- Standard 1: Motor skills and movement patterns, 1A, 1B, 1C, 1E, 1F
- Standard 2: Movement concepts and principles, 2D

### Table 2.3 Summary of Wellness Week 3 Activities

| Activity | Day 1 Monday | Day 2 Tuesday | Day 3 Wednesday | Day 4 Thursday | Day 5 Friday |
|---|---|---|---|---|---|
| Morning Activity Break | Video routine performed every day of the week: Wave It | | | | |
| Daily Message | Get your muscles ready. | Move your body. | Food for strong bones and muscles | You have only one body; make it fit! | If it is to be, it's up to me. |
| Afternoon Activity Break | If You're Happy and You Know It | Pattern Practice | Simon Says | Follow the Leader | Shoe Color Lineup |
| Eat Well Wednesday Classroom Discussion | — | — | Fuel Up: Foods With Protein | — | — |
| Schoolwide Events | — | — | Eat Well Wednesday: Fuel Up: Yogurt Bar in the Cafeteria | — | Get Fit Friday: TEAM Time 3: Little Kids Lead |

- Standard 3: Participates in physical activity, 3A, 3B, 3C
- Standard 4: Achieves health-enhancing physical fitness, 4A, 4B, 4C, 4D, 4E
- Standard 5: Exhibits responsible behavior and respect for others, 5A, 5B, 5C, 5G, 5H
- Standard 6: Values physical activity for health and social interactions, 6A, 6B, 6C, 6G

## Week 3 Math Standards

For specific focal points see appendix B.

- Numbers and operations (counting with understanding, ordinal and cardinal numbers)
- Algebra (sort, classify, order, sequence, pattern, add, subtract)
- Measurement (measure units, select units and tools, measure in units using measurement tools)
- Data analysis and probability (represent data using concrete objects, pictures, and graphs)

## Week 3 Standards for Other Curriculum Areas

Standards for other academic areas, such as sciences and language arts, were considered in developing lessons. Appendix B includes the sources of these standards.

## Week 3 Resources

There are three types of printed resources for use in Wellness Week 3: signs, worksheets, and newsletters. Web-based resources are also provided.

### Signs

General signs (described in more detail on page 17) can be used during Wellness Week 3 and reused in subsequent Wellness Weeks. Other signs are specifically for use during Wellness Week 3.

 **General**

G1: Fitness for Life: Elementary School

G2: Wellness Week

G3: Physical Activity Pyramid for Kids

G4: MyPyramid for Kids

G5: Eat Well Wednesday

G6: TEAM Time: Together Everyone Achieves More

G7: Get Fit Friday

G8: Healthy mind, healthy body, healthy heart . . . let's start!

G9: ABCs of Physical Activity

G10: ABCs of Nutrition

 **Wellness Week 3 → Signs**

3.1: Physical Activity Pyramid: Do exercise for muscle fitness and flexibility!

*3.2: Before you play or perform, you need to get your muscles warm!

3.3: Music helps you move!

3.4: Blue is for milk; purple is for meat and beans!

*3.5: Protein power! Get strong, live long!

*3.6: We have only one body. Let's make it fit!

3.7: One rule of fitness you need to know: Challenging your muscles makes them grow!

*3.8: If it is to be, it's up to me!

---

* Indicates signs used for chants

### Worksheets

The DVD includes black-and-white versions of all Week 3 signs that you can print and use

> ★ **teacher tip • • •**
> Choose a bulletin board to use for wellness in your classroom. During each Wellness Week, post the general signs all week. Each day of Wellness Week, feature the signs of the day, or post all daily signs and point out the sign of the day on appropriate days. If possible, feature the sign of the day at the front of the classroom. At the end of Wellness Week, continue to feature wellness on the wellness bulletin board, rotating signs from time to time.

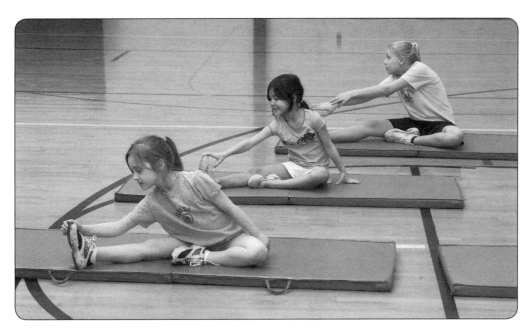

Lessons and messages in Wellness Week 3 emphasize flexibility and muscle fitness.

as coloring worksheets. In addition, the DVD includes black-and-white versions of MyPyramid for Kids and the Physical Activity Pyramid for Kids for coloring.

 **Wellness Week 3 → Worksheets**

## Newsletters

The DVD contains a newsletter for use during each Wellness Week. It is recommended that your wellness coordinator edit, print, and distribute these newsletters. If you do not have a wellness coordinator, or if your coordinator does not handle the newsletters, you can do it yourself. Just open the appropriate newsletter file, follow the instructions to edit and customize the newsletter, print it, and distribute it, either electronically or by sending copies home with the students. Remind students to talk to their families about Wellness Week and the information in the newsletters.

 **Wellness Week 3 → Newsletter**

## Web Resources

Available at www.mypyramid.gov: a My-Pyramid worksheet and nutrition activities

Available at www.dole.com/superkids/: *Kids Cookbook*, games, puzzles, and other nutrition activities

# Week 3 Special Days

Each Wellness Week, two schoolwide activities are featured. On Eat Well Wednesday, nutrition is the focus, and on Get Fit Friday, physical activity is the focus. These activities provide opportunities for the whole school to have a common experience and to highlight the importance of nutrition and physical activity to health and wellness.

## Eat Well Wednesday

During each Wellness Week, Day 3 (typically Wednesday) is known as Eat Well Wednesday. On this day, teachers and staff are encouraged to emphasize the weekly nutrition message. Special schoolwide events (e.g., a lunch salad bar or healthy snack preparation) may be planned by the wellness coordinator. Teachers are encouraged to support these Eat Well Wednesday events and plan special Eat Well Wednesday events in their classrooms, emphasizing sound nutrition. During Wellness Week 3, a yogurt bar will be set up in the cafeteria.

WEEK 3 • INTRODUCTION

## Get Fit Friday

During each Wellness Week, Day 5 (typically Friday) is known as Get Fit Friday. On this day, a schoolwide event focusing on physical activity will be planned by the wellness coordinator. The Get Fit Friday activities are called TEAM Time activities (TEAM stands for Together Everyone Achieves More).

During Wellness Week 3, the TEAM Time activity planned for Get Fit Friday is called Little Kids Lead. The wellness coordinator and students from kindergarten, first grade, and second grade will lead all students in three different activities. First, kindergarten students will lead an activity called We Get Fit, then first-grade students will lead an activity called CYIM Fit, and finally second-grade students will lead an activity called Wave It. These activities will have been learned in physical education or in the classroom earlier in the week.

## USING THE VIDEO ACTIVITIES

During each Wellness Week, you will play an activity video every day. The five videos use the same activity routine but present different conceptual messages for each day of the week. Simply play the appropriate video and have your students perform the routine for that day. The DVD also provides an instructional video for each week's routine. If your school has a physical education teacher, he or she may have taught the routine to students during the week before Wellness Week, in which case you won't have to use the instructional video. Otherwise, you can use it to help your students learn the routine.

In the instructional video, the instructor faces away from your students for some of the left–right movements. Explain to students that they should do those movements the same way the instructor does them. That is, when the instructor moves to the right, they should also move to the right. However, in the daily activity videos, the leaders face forward, so their left–right movements are in reverse (mirror image). While following along with the daily activity videos, your students should move in the opposite direction of the leaders for left–right movements. Keep in mind that although moving in the correct direction is desirable, the key is to get all kids moving regardless of the direction. If your students have a hard time performing the activity, feel free to replay the instructional video.

WEEK 3 • INTRODUCTION

## Day 1 Lesson Plan

## OVERVIEW

* **Morning Activity Break**: Wave It (DVD routine)
* **Afternoon Activity Break**: If You're Happy and You Know It

## OBJECTIVES

Students will

* participate in 10 minutes of moderate to vigorous physical activity;
* when asked, repeat the message that it's good to warm up their muscles by moving slowly before they move fast;
* list two activities that make their muscles stronger; and
* participate in physical activity, making only supportive comments to themselves and others.

## RESOURCES

### Signs

 **General**

G2: Wellness Week

G3: Physical Activity Pyramid for Kids

G8: Healthy mind, healthy body, healthy heart . . . let's start!

 **Wellness Week 3 → Signs**

3.1: Physical Activity Pyramid: Do exercise for muscle fitness and flexibility!

* 3.2: Before you play or perform, you need to get your muscles warm!

---

\* Indicates sign used for chant

### Worksheets

The DVD includes black-and-white versions of today's signs that you can print and use as coloring worksheets. In addition, the DVD includes black-and-white versions of MyPyramid for Kids and the Physical Activity Pyramid for Kids for coloring.

 **Wellness Week 3 → Worksheets**

# MORNING ACTIVITY BREAK

**DVD Routine**: Wave It

## Introduction

"It's important to be physically active every day. This week we're going to be talking about getting stronger. When we use our bodies, the muscles get stronger. In our routine we are going to use all the different parts of our bodies, so lots of different parts will get stronger. It's always important to warm up our muscles by moving around at medium speed before we stretch them or move fast."

> ⭐ **teacher tip • • •**
> Your enthusiasm will go a long way to "sell" physical activity as an important part of daily life. Focus on enjoying this active time yourself as well as on the importance of it for your children's minds and bodies!

## Video Routine

The DVD has five versions of the Wave It routine, one for each day of the week. It also has a special instructional version that teaches students how to do the routine.

1. Play the instructional routine. If the PE teacher has already taught the routine to the students, you can skip this step.
2. Play the Day 1 routine.

Each day the current version of the routine promotes a new and different message. Variations on the message play before the first routine, between routines, and after the last routine. For Wave It, the Day 1 message is "Get your muscles ready," and the three variations are as follows:

✳ You need to get your muscles warm before you play or perform. Start moving slowly, then move fast—now your muscles are ready to last.

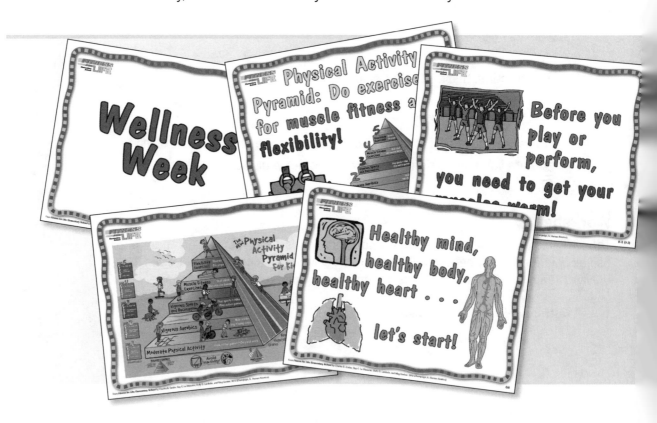

WEEK **3** • DAY **1**

* You need to get your muscles warm before you play or perform. Start moving slowly, then move fast—now your muscles are ready to last.
* Warm up before you exercise because it will help your muscles stretch farther. Warm muscles allow you to jump higher, reach farther, and run faster.

> **? comprehension check • • •**
> "Point to your movement space. That's right, move in just one place, not around the room."
>
> "Before we start, let's go over a special signal. When I clap my hands like this"—clap your hands three times, or choose your own attention signal—"I want you to stop moving and look at me. Let's practice. Start marching in place. (Clap, clap, clap.) You did a great job stopping and looking right at me."

## Breathing

After finishing the routine, lead the class in breathing.

> **👁 observation • • •**
> We're talking about muscular strength and flexibility this week. Look for examples of the major muscle groups the students are using. Are their legs or arms getting tired? That's a great sign that they are getting stronger. Tell them so.

"Breathing deeply is important for our bodies, so we'll end every activity with a couple of deep breaths. Let's all breathe in deeply (count 1, 2), hold (count 1, 2), breathe out (count 1, 2), and hold (count 1, 2)." Repeat three times.

## Background Information

* Starting slowly when we move helps warm up our muscles—it's good to walk a bit, jog a bit, and then start to run.
* Muscles are smart. They have little sensors in them, and if we don't alert the sensors by warming up, sometimes they can make it more difficult to move well.

## Discussion

* "Your muscles can stretch farther when they are warm. Being able to stretch farther is called flexibility. Do you know anything else that gets more flexible when it gets warm?"
* "When you use your muscles a lot, they get stronger. Point to muscles that you used today in our routine."
* "What muscles do you use a lot? Which of your muscles are strong?"

## Chant

Chanting is a great way to reinforce messages. If you've posted the corresponding sign, point to it, and tell the students that when you say the first phrase, they should respond by saying the second phrase. Use any of your favorite chants from past lessons as well as the new one for today. Make it fun!

Teacher: "Before you play or perform . . ."

Students: ". . . you need to get your muscles warm!"

Practice several times until the students respond easily to your prompt.

## Closure

Closure provides an opportunity to focus one more time on the main message of the lesson by using compliments, reviewing messages, and making suggestions for doing activity at home. Closure also includes a brief preview of what's coming in the next lesson to help students see connections and begin to prepare for future lessons.

### Compliments

"You did a great job following the video and got some exercise for your arms and legs and hips."

> ↻ **review** • • •
> "When you've been working hard, your muscles feel different. Take a moment and just notice how your muscles feel. This is what it feels like when they are growing stronger. It happens in the quiet time after you exercise, when your muscles are resting. Today we talked about starting slowly to warm up our muscles and how using our muscles makes us stronger."

### Take It Home

"What kinds of activities do you do at home that can make your muscles stronger? What kinds of activities could you do? Whom could you ask to join you in those activities?"

### Preview

"Since this is Wellness Week, we're really going to try to be especially active. We're going to take a break like this and enjoy time moving every day."

## AFTERNOON ACTIVITY BREAK

**Activity**: If You're Happy and You Know It

Perform in the afternoon or at some other time during the day when the students need a physical activity break.

Teach children the song and motions to "If you're happy and you know it, clap your hands."

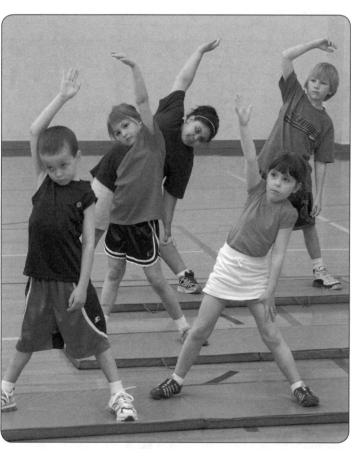

Before you exercise, warm up your muscles.

✳ If you're happy and you know it, clap your hands.

✳ If you're happy and you know it, clap your hands.

✳ If you're happy and you know it, then your face will surely show it.

✳ If you're happy and you know it, clap your hands.

Add movement verses such as the following, or make up your own.

✳ March in place.
✳ Stand and sit.
✳ Wave your hands.
✳ Jump in place.
✳ Shake a hand.
✳ Run in place.

### Breathing

After finishing the activity, lead the class in breathing.

"Breathing deeply is important for our bodies, so we'll end every activity with a couple of deep breaths. Let's all breathe in deeply (count 1, 2), hold (count 1, 2), breathe out (count 1, 2), and hold (count 1, 2)." Repeat three times.

## Closure

"Thanks for showing such good body control. You all did that without any problems even though we are in a small space. Since you have such good body control,

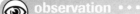

**observation** • • •

Students are encouraged to stay in their own play space by their desks. Look for signs of body control and good use of space. Prompt when necessary, and compliment them on their control if appropriate.

we'll be able to do lots of fun things because I won't have to worry about you getting hurt when you are moving in this little space."

## ADDITIONAL ACTIVITIES

See appendix A for additional enriching and integrative outdoor activities. For more information, go to www.fitnessforlife.org.

WEEK **3** • DAY **1**

# 3 WELLNESS WEEK

## Day 2 Lesson Plan

### OVERVIEW

* **Morning Activity Break**: Wave It (DVD routine)
* **Afternoon Activity Break**: Pattern Practice

### OBJECTIVES

Students will

* participate in 10 minutes of moderate to vigorous physical activity;
* when asked, repeat the message that music helps them enjoy moving;
* participate in physical activity, making only supportive comments to themselves and others; and
* identify the correct movement to continue an ABCD pattern, and perform the pattern of movements.

### RESOURCES

#### Signs

 **Wellness Week 3 → Signs**

3.3: Music helps you move!

#### Worksheets

The DVD includes a black-and-white version of today's sign that you can print and use as a coloring worksheet. In addition, the DVD includes black-and-white versions of MyPyramid for Kids and the Physical Activity Pyramid for Kids for coloring.

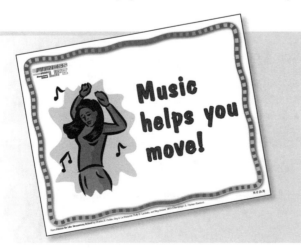

Music helps you move!

 **Wellness Week 3 → Worksheets**

### MORNING ACTIVITY BREAK

**DVD Routine**: Wave It

#### Introduction

"Yesterday we talked about how important it is to start slowly and warm up our muscles before moving fast. This week we are talking about helping our muscles get stronger and stretching them to be more flexible. When our muscles are warm, we can move farther at each joint. It is good to strengthen our muscles and to stretch them. This song helps us to do that to a good beat."

## Video Routine

The DVD has five versions of the Wave It routine, one for each day of the week. It also has a special instructional version that teaches students how to do the routine.

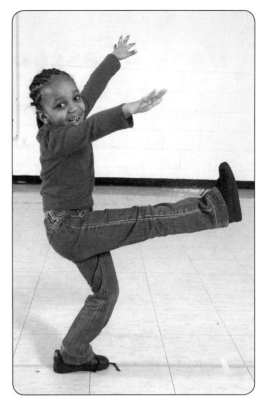

1. If the students have not done this week's routine before, play the instructional routine. If the PE teacher has already taught the routine to the students, or if they have already practiced the instructional routine with you, you can skip this step.

2. Play the Day 2 routine.

Each day the current version of the routine promotes a new and different message. Variations on the message play before the first routine, between routines, and after the last routine. For Wave It, the Day 2 message is "Move your body," and the three variations are as follows:

＊ You have many body parts to move. Move with the music; get in the groove.

＊ To move to the music, you need quick feet; keep your body moving to the beat.

＊ Singing and moving with friends are fun. You'll move all of your body before you're done.

Moving your body parts in different ways is fun, especially when you're moving to the beat of music.

## Breathing

After finishing the routine, lead the class in breathing.

"Breathing deeply is important for our bodies, so we'll end every activity with a couple of deep breaths. Let's all breathe in deeply (count 1, 2), hold (count 1, 2), breathe out (count 1, 2), and hold (count 1, 2)." Repeat three times.

## Background Information

＊ Moving with friends makes whatever you do fun.

＊ The beat of the music helps you move. Fast music makes it easier to move faster; slow music makes it easier to move slowly.

＊ Music can make you happy and make time pass quickly.

## Discussion

＊ "Name one body part you moved in the song."

＊ "Does having the music play help you to keep moving?"

＊ "What other things help you to keep moving?" (e.g., doing it with a friend or movements you like to do—like skipping)

> **teacher tip • • •**
> Chanting can be fun and really help remind us of important points. Be enthusiastic, use different accents, and sometimes allow the students to shout back their responses. Encourage students to teach the chants to their families.

WEEK **3** • DAY **2**

## Chant

Chanting is a great way to reinforce messages. If you've posted the corresponding sign, point to it, and tell the students that when you say the first phrase, they should respond by saying the second phrase. Use the chant from the Day 1 lesson or any other chants that you like from previous lessons. Make it fun!

> Teacher: "Before you play or perform . . ."
>
> Students: ". . . you need to get your muscles warm!"

Practice several times until the students respond easily to your prompt.

## Closure

Closure provides an opportunity to focus one more time on the main message of the lesson by using compliments, reviewing messages, and making suggestions for doing activity at home. Closure also includes a brief preview of what's coming in the next lesson to help students see connections and begin to prepare for future lessons.

### Compliments

"You did a great job following the video. There were lots of directions to follow in the song—up and down, left and right. You were listening and getting better and better at moving to the beat. Moving to the beat is fun."

🔄 review • • •
"Today we talked about strengthening and stretching our muscles and about moving to the beat. When you move your arms a lot, do they get tired? Do they feel stronger? Usually they will be tired when you stop, but stronger the next day."

### Take It Home

"When you are at home, put on some music and ask someone to move with you to the beat."

### Preview

"Tomorrow we'll get even stronger and find some new ways to line up."

## AFTERNOON ACTIVITY BREAK

**Activity**: Pattern Practice

Perform in the afternoon or at some other time during the day when the students need a physical activity break.

✖️ interdisciplinary • • •
This activity helps children practice patterns in movement. Being able to recognize, follow, and create patterns are also important skills in math.

"A pattern is something we do over and over the same way. Remember when we did an ABAB pattern like stand up, sit down, stand up, sit down? Then we did an ABC pattern. How many movements did it have? Right, three! One for A, one for B, and one for C. Today we are going to do an ABCD pattern. How many movements do you think it will need? Right, four. Let's make A stand for stand up, B for jump, C for clap, and D for sit down. Let's do that all together. Stand up, jump, clap, sit down. To repeat the pattern, what do we do next? Right! Stand up, jump, clap, sit down. Let's do it five times together." (If you want to try other ABCD patterns, try stand up, clap, jump, sit down.)

Write the pattern on the board. Talk about patterns, how to extend them, and how you can look at them in different ways: as single units, as groups of units, and so on. For instance, A B C D = AB CD.

## Breathing

After finishing the activity, lead the class in breathing.

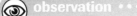

**observation** • • •

We're talking about muscular strength and flexibility this week. Look for examples of the major muscle groups the students are using. Are their legs or arms getting tired? That's a great sign that they are getting stronger. Tell them so.

"Breathing deeply is important for our bodies, so we'll end every activity with a couple of deep breaths. Let's all breathe in deeply (count 1, 2), hold (count 1, 2), breathe out (count 1, 2), and hold (count 1, 2)." Repeat three times.

## Closure

"Wow, you're great at patterns. You did a four-part pattern. We can make up lots of patterns to do. It just takes practice to get good at them. Thanks for showing such good body control. You all did that without any problems even though we are in a small space. Since you have such good body control, we can keep doing active games in the classroom. I won't have to worry about you getting hurt when you are moving in this little space."

## ADDITIONAL ACTIVITIES

See appendix A for additional enriching and integrative outdoor activities. For more information, go to www.fitnessforlife.org.

WEEK **3** • DAY **2**

# 3 WELLNESS WEEK

## Day 3 Lesson Plan ••••••••••••••••••••••••••

### OVERVIEW

* **Morning Activity Break**: Wave It (DVD routine)
* **Eat Well Wednesday Class Discussion**: Fuel Up: Foods With Protein
* **Eat Well Wednesday Activity**: Fuel Up: Yogurt Bar in the Cafeteria
* **Afternoon Activity Break**: Simon Says

### OBJECTIVES

Students will

* participate in 10 minutes of moderate to vigorous physical activity,
* repeat (correctly) the message that certain foods build strong bones and muscles,
* name two foods that build strong bones and muscles,
* practice decision making and attention by responding with movement on appropriate verbal cues (Simon Says) and not responding when the cue is missing,
* identify the color stripe on the food pyramid representing protein (blue), and
* understand that protein is vital for cell repair and muscle growth.

### RESOURCES

#### Signs

 **General**

G4: MyPyramid for Kids
G5: Eat Well Wednesday
G10: ABCs of Nutrition

 **Wellness Week 3 → Signs**

3.4: Blue is for milk; purple is for meat and beans!
* 3.5: Protein power! Get strong, live long!

---

* Indicates sign used for chant

#### Worksheets

The DVD includes black-and-white versions of today's signs that you can print and use as coloring worksheets. In addition, the DVD includes black-and-white versions of MyPyramid for Kids and the Physical Activity Pyramid for Kids for coloring.

 **Wellness Week 3 → Worksheets**

WEEK 3 • DAY 3

## Web Resources

Consider activities from www.mypyramid.gov, www.dole.com/superkids/, or http://fueluptoplay60.com/about-fuel-up-to-play.html.

# MORNING ACTIVITY BREAK

**DVD Routine**: Wave It

## Introduction

"Wellness Week reminds us of things we should be doing every week and every day. Yesterday we talked about how music helps us keep moving. We've also talked about how moving makes us stronger and stretching makes us more flexible. Today we'll talk about foods that make our bones and muscles strong. Doing the routine should be easier today because this is our third day trying it. Show me your good body control again today."

## Video Routine

The DVD has five versions of the Wave It routine, one for each day of the week. It also has a special instructional version that teaches students how to do the routine.

1. If the students have not done this week's routine before, play the instructional routine. If the PE teacher has already taught the routine to the students, or if they have already practiced the instructional routine with you, you can skip this step.

2. Play the Day 3 routine.

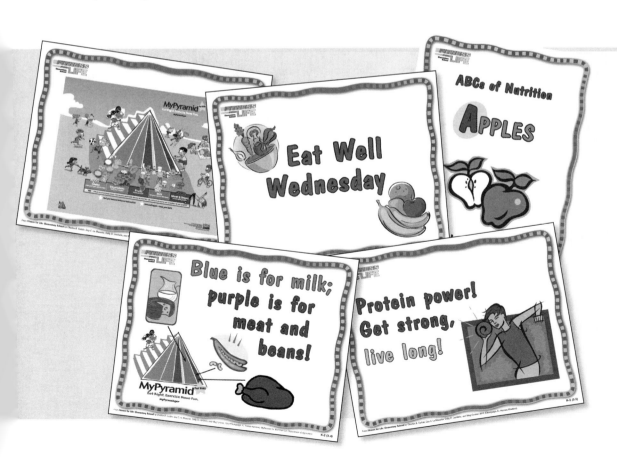

WEEK 3 · DAY 3

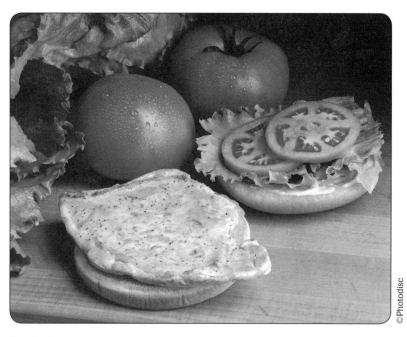

©Photodisc

Foods that provide calcium and protein help build strong bones and muscles.

Each day the current version of the routine promotes a new and different message. Variations on the message play before the first routine, between routines, and after the last routine. For Wave It, the Day 3 message is "Food for strong bones and muscles," and the three variations are as follows:

❋ Strong bones, strong muscles, strong teeth—yes, please! Let's drink milk and eat beans and a little cheese.

❋ Eggs and fish and vegetable greens build muscles and bones like you've never seen.

❋ Our muscles get protein from beans, meat, milk, cheese, and eggs. Our bones get calcium from milk, cheese, and green leafy vegetables. Eat some of these foods every day to grow strong and play.

### observation • • •

Look around the room. Are the children showing good body control? Are there any parts of the routine that are particularly hard, creating stumbling blocks for the students? Note any problems so you can have the students practice that piece, or you can modify the routine to allow them to flow through it.

### Breathing

After finishing the routine, lead the class in breathing.

"Breathing deeply is important for our bodies, so we'll end every activity with a couple of deep breaths. Let's all breathe in deeply (count 1, 2), hold (count 1, 2), breathe out (count 1, 2), and hold (count 1, 2)." Repeat three times.

### Background Information

❋ Protein helps build muscles; calcium helps build strong bones.

❋ Every cell in the body contains protein.

❋ Some foods are very high in protein and help build muscles—fish, tofu, beef, chicken, and eggs.

❋ Some foods are very high in calcium and help build bones—milk, cheese, and green leafy vegetables.

❋ When choosing meat as part of a diet, choose lean cuts that have less fat.

### Discussion

❋ "How many glasses of milk do you drink each day? Do you drink one at breakfast or have it on your cereal? Do you drink milk at lunch? In the afternoon? At supper? Count for yourself. Show me on your fingers. Try to drink three glasses of milk each day. Milk helps build strong bones."

WEEK 3 • DAY 3

✳ "Name some foods that have protein that you eat at home or at school."

✳ "Can you name a dark leafy vegetable (e.g., spinach, kale, collard greens)? These foods also help build strong bones."

## Chant

Chanting is a great way to reinforce messages. If you've posted the corresponding sign, point to it, and tell the students that when you say the first phrase, they should respond by saying the second phrase. Make it fun!

Teacher: "Protein power! Get strong . . ."

Students: ". . . live long!"

Practice several times until the students respond easily to your prompt.

## Closure

Closure provides an opportunity to focus one more time on the main message of the lesson by using compliments, reviewing messages, and making suggestions for doing activity at home. Closure also includes a brief preview of what's coming in the next lesson to help students see connections and begin to prepare for future lessons.

### *Compliments*

"You did lots of good exercising while singing Wave It. I saw lots of great stretching and lots of bending and straightening. You helped make your muscles strong and your body flexible."

### *Take It Home*

"Ask if you can go along on a grocery shopping trip and look for dark green veggies at the store."

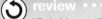 **review** • • •

"Drinking milk and eating cheese, fish, beans, and dark green veggies make your bones and muscles strong. Which of those do you remember drinking or eating?"

### *Preview*

"Tomorrow we're going to talk about getting fit."

# EAT WELL WEDNESDAY

Each Wednesday all teachers and staff are encouraged to emphasize the weekly nutrition message. Special schoolwide events (e.g., a lunch salad bar or healthy snack preparation) may be planned by the wellness coordinator. Teachers are encouraged to support these Eat Well Wednesday events and plan special Eat Well Wednesday events in their classrooms, emphasizing sound nutrition.

## Eat Well Wednesday Class Discussion

**Nutrition Topic:** Fuel Up: Foods With Protein

### *Introduction*

Introduce MyPyramid and the healthy food groups of the week: milk, and meat and beans (foods with protein). MyPyramid is a guideline for healthy eating, introducing the five food groups (plus oils): grains, vegetables, fruits, milk, and meat and beans. Each food group represents a different nutrition category.

### Background Information

✳ When you treat your body well, it will grow, keep itself strong, and heal itself when hurt. Nutrients are elements in healthy foods with special jobs. There are six nutrient types (carbohydrate, vitamins, minerals, fat, protein, and water). By eating a wide variety of foods, every color every day, your body receives all the nutrients it needs to learn, move, and grow.

✳ Protein is an important source of energy used to repair cells, build muscles, and help the body grow.

✳ Protein comes from nuts, meat, beans, fish, and dairy foods like milk, yogurt, and cheese.

✳ Eating healthy snacks during the school day fuels the brain for learning.

✳ One serving of yogurt can provide 10 to 20 percent of daily protein needs.

### Discussion

✳ "What are some snacks that are energy rich?" (For instance, yogurt and nuts contain protein.)

✳ "What are some snacks that are energy poor?" (For example, potato chips contain lots of salt and fat.)

✳ "Can we name different foods we eat that contain protein?"

✳ "Let's list what we ate today and think about which foods contained lots of protein."

This week have your students prepare and eat healthy snacks to make sure their bodies are receiving all the nutrients they need to learn, move, and grow (e.g., celery with peanut butter and raisins or apple slices with peanut butter).

### Take It Home

✳ "Find out the favorite energy-rich snack of a family member."

✳ "With your family, plan an energy-rich snack for after school each day and to bring to school for healthy snacks during the week."

## Eat Well Wednesday Schoolwide Activity

During Wellness Week 3, a yogurt bar will be set up in the cafeteria.

## AFTERNOON ACTIVITY BREAK

**Activity**: Simon Says

Perform in the afternoon or at other times when the students need a physical activity break.

Begin by explaining how the game works. Tell them that when you start an instruction with "Simon says," they should do what you say. But if you simply tell them to do something, such as "Wave your arms," they shouldn't respond. Then lead them through several examples so they understand how the game works. For instance, if you say, "Simon says, 'Put your hands on your hips,'" the students should put their hands on their hips. But if you say, "Jump up and

**⊗ interdisciplinary • • •**

This activity includes movement and helps students practice categorizing skills since they have to put the instructions into one of two categories: instructions to follow and instructions to ignore. The activity also provides practice in number operations by using various methods for defining the number of times to do each movement.

down three times," they should stay still because you didn't say, "Simon says". If the students make mistakes, don't worry; just go on to the next action.

**? comprehension check • • •**

"Show me what you will do if I say, 'Simon says, "Touch your shoulders."' Show me what you will do if I say, 'Touch your knees' without saying, 'Simon says.'"

You can use number operations when telling the students the number of times to do something (e.g., instead of saying four times, use two plus two). Have students use addition, subtraction, less than, more than, and so on to determine the number of times to do each exercise.

If students make mistakes just say "Oops," laugh with them, and then go on with the next action. Include lots of flexing and extending, and bending and stretching since this week we are talking about strengthening and stretching muscles. (Some suggested activities: bend and straighten elbows; sit down, stand up; up on toes; stand on heels with toes up; run in place; reach high with one hand, reach high with the other; twist.) End with more gentle movements so the students gradually calm down, and the heart slows down.

**◉ observation • • •**

We're talking about muscular strength and flexibility this week. Look for examples of the major muscle groups the students are using. Are their legs or arms getting tired? That's a great sign that they are getting stronger. Tell them so.

## Breathing

After finishing the activity, lead the class in breathing.

"Breathing deeply is important for our bodies, so we'll end every activity with a couple of deep breaths. Let's all breathe in deeply (count 1, 2), hold (count 1, 2), breathe out (count 1, 2), and hold (count 1, 2)." Repeat three times.

## Closure

"Thanks for showing such good body control. You paid careful attention to what Simon said to do. That's careful listening. Careful listening helps you learn lots of new things. You also helped get your muscles stronger and your body more flexible."

# ADDITIONAL ACTIVITIES

See appendix A for additional enriching and integrative outdoor activities. For more information, go to www.fitnessforlife.org.

WEEK 3 • DAY 3

# Day 4 Lesson Plan

## OVERVIEW

* **Morning Activity Break**: Wave It (DVD routine)
* **Afternoon Activity Break**: Follow the Leader

## OBJECTIVES

Students will

* participate in 10 minutes of moderate to vigorous physical activity;
* repeat the message that doing a little more even when they are tired helps their muscles get stronger; and
* participate in physical activity, making only supportive comments to themselves and others.

## RESOURCES

### Signs

 **Wellness Week 3 → Signs**

* 3.6: We have only one body. Let's make it fit!

  3.7: One rule of fitness you need to know: Challenging your muscles makes them grow!

* Indicates sign used for chant

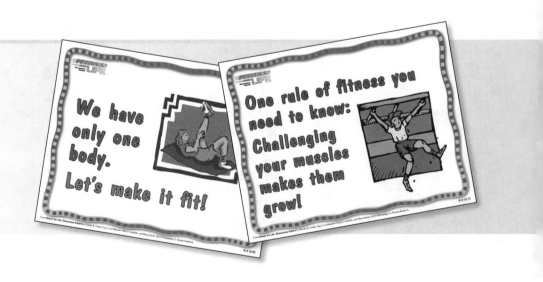

## Worksheets

The DVD includes black-and-white versions of today's signs that you can print and use as coloring worksheets. In addition, the DVD includes black-and-white versions of MyPyramid for Kids and the Physical Activity Pyramid for Kids for coloring.

 **Wellness Week 3 → Worksheets**

# MORNING ACTIVITY BREAK

**DVD Routine**: Wave It

## Introduction

"Yesterday we talked about foods that help your bones and muscles be strong. The right foods and good activity help you get stronger. If you do a little more than you are used to, it really helps your muscles."

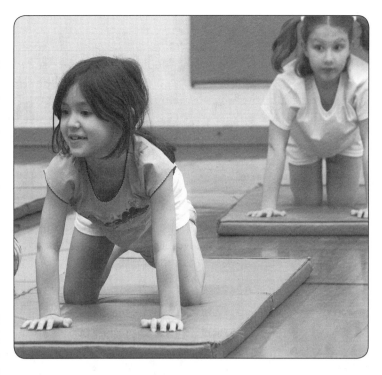

Challenge the muscles to make them grow and help make the body fit.

## Video Routine

The DVD has five versions of the Wave It routine, one for each day of the week. It also has a special instructional version that teaches students how to do the routine.

1. If the students have not done this week's routine before, play the instructional routine. If the PE teacher has already taught the routine to the students, or if they have already practiced the instructional routine with you, you can skip this step.
2. Play the Day 4 routine.

Each day the current version of the routine promotes a new and different message. Variations on the message play before the first routine, between routines, and after the last routine. For Wave It, the Day 4 message is "You have only one body; make it fit," and the three variations are as follows:

* One rule of fitness you need to know: challenging your muscles makes them grow.
* *Overload* means doing more than you usually do. It's a basic rule of fitness that applies to me and you.
* Take care of your body and exercise a lot; it's the only one you've got. Be a responsible body owner; take good care of your one and only body.

> **observation** • • •
> Look around the room. Are the students doing the activity with ease? Tell them how well they are doing and how much better they have gotten with practice.

WEEK **3** • DAY **4**

## Breathing

After finishing the routine, lead the class in breathing.

"Breathing deeply is important for our bodies, so we'll end every activity with a couple of deep breaths. Let's all breathe in deeply (count 1, 2), hold (count 1, 2), breathe out (count 1, 2), and hold (count 1, 2)." Repeat three times.

## Background Information

❋ When your body is healthy and fit, you feel better and have more energy.

❋ Being responsible means taking care of things. Your body is a good thing to take care of, and you do this by choosing healthy foods, getting rest, and being physically active.

❋ For muscles to get stronger they need to be used. If you do a little more than you have done before, your muscle responds by getting stronger. This is called overloading the muscle.

## Discussion

❋ "Who is responsible for taking care of your body?"

❋ "Who decides whether to watch TV or be physically active?"

❋ "Have you ever been tired and wanted to stop moving, but then just pushed yourself a little more to keep going? That was a time when your muscles got stronger!"

## Chant

Chanting is a great way to reinforce messages. If you've posted the corresponding sign, point to it, and tell the students that when you say the first phrase, they should respond by saying the second phrase. Make it fun!

Teacher: "We have only one body."

Students: "Let's make it fit!"

Practice several times until the students respond easily to your prompt.

## Closure

Closure provides an opportunity to focus one more time on the main message of the lesson by using compliments, reviewing messages, and making suggestions for doing activity at home. Closure also includes a brief preview of what's coming in the next lesson to help students see connections and begin to prepare for future lessons.

### *Compliments*

"You're getting so good at the routine that it looks like you can almost do it without thinking about it. You are getting good enough to sing or hum along as you are doing it. It's hard to do that when you are first learning the routine. Your practice has helped you learn the routine so you don't have to concentrate on it so much anymore."

### *Take It Home*

"When someone asks you to help with something at home, like

**review** • • •

"Think about how your muscles feel when you've been moving around a lot. Can you describe the feeling? Next time you feel your muscles are tired, you can know that is a good thing. When you are tired, doing a little more makes you stronger."

cleaning or taking out the trash, and you are tired, do you think you could push yourself to do a little more because you know it will help you get stronger?"

### Preview

"Tomorrow we'll do Wave It and be better than ever!"

# AFTERNOON ACTIVITY BREAK

**Activity**: Follow the Leader

Perform in the afternoon or at some other time during the day when the students need a physical activity break.

Begin by telling the students, "In Follow the Leader you do just what I do. Ready? Here we go." Start with simple actions; for example, put your hands in the air and wave them back and forth. Try to do at least 8 counts of each movement. So you might march in place and count 1, 2, 3, 4, 5, 6, 7, 8; clap your hands 1, 2, 3, 4, 5, 6, 7, 8; or run in place. You can also count to 30 by doing 3 movements 10 times each. Talk about counting and explain that 3 sets of 10 equals 30.

Since we are talking about getting stronger and more flexible, put in lots of standing up, sitting down, stretching, and bending and straightening joints. You may even add some push-ups or animal walks. Let the children suggest their favorites. When you get near the end, do slower movements to allow their hearts to slow down again. Tell them you are doing this.

## Breathing

After finishing the activity, lead the class in breathing.

"Breathing deeply is important for our bodies. so we'll end every

activity with a couple of deep breaths. Let's all breathe in deeply (count 1, 2), hold (count 1, 2), breathe out (count 1, 2), and hold (count 1, 2)." Repeat three times.

## Closure

"You worked hard today and used lots of muscles. Yesterday you paid careful attention to what Simon said. Today you worked hard and paid careful attention to what I was doing. That's careful watching. Being able to watch carefully and copy what you see helps you learn lots of skills."

# ADDITIONAL ACTIVITIES

See appendix A for additional enriching and integrative outdoor activities. For more information, go to www.fitnessforlife.org.

WEEK **3** • DAY **4**

# 3 WELLNESS WEEK

## Day 5 Lesson Plan

## OVERVIEW

* **Get Fit Friday Activity:** TEAM Time 3: Little Kids Lead
* **Morning Activity Break**: Wave It (DVD routine)
* **Afternoon Activity Break**: Shoe Color Lineup

## OBJECTIVES

Students will

* participate in 10 minutes of moderate to vigorous physical activity;
* move fluidly and confidently during the video routine;
* repeat the message that the secret to success is trying;
* participate in physical activity, making only supportive comments to themselves and others; and
* be team members who try to help the team accomplish the task (Shoe Color Lineup).

## RESOURCES

### Signs

 **General**

> G6: TEAM Time: Together Everyone Achieves More
> G7: Get Fit Friday

 **Wellness Week 3 → Signs**

> * 3.8: If it is to be, it's up to me!

―――――――――

\* Indicates sign used for chant

### Worksheets

The DVD includes a black-and-white version of today's sign that you can print and use as a coloring worksheet. In addition, the DVD includes black-and-white versions of MyPyramid for Kids and the Physical Activity Pyramid for Kids for coloring.

 **Wellness Week 3 → Worksheets**

## GET FIT FRIDAY

During each Wellness Week, Day 5 (typically Friday) is known as Get Fit Friday. On this day, a schoolwide event focusing on physical activity will be planned by the wellness coordinator. The Get Fit Friday activities are called TEAM Time activities (TEAM stands for Together Everyone Achieves More).

During Wellness Week 3, the TEAM Time activity planned for Get Fit Friday is called Little Kids Lead. The wellness coordinator and students from kindergarten, first grade, and second grade will lead all students in three different activities. First, kindergarten students will lead an activity called We Get Fit, then first-grade students will lead an activity called CYIM Fit, and finally second-grade students will lead an activity called Wave It. These activities will have been learned in physical education or in the classroom earlier in the week.

In addition to supporting Little Kids Lead, mention the TEAM Time activity as you discuss the video routine messages during the morning activity break.

# MORNING ACTIVITY BREAK

**DVD Routine**: Wave It

## Introduction

"We've been doing the Wave It video all week, so today we should be getting pretty good at it. I hope you can sing or hum along as you do it. Try it. Trying hard means paying attention to what you are doing, but when you have done that a lot, and you get really good, sometimes you can do it without even having to think about it. Let's see if we can do this routine easily."

## Video Routine

The DVD has five versions of the Wave It routine, one for each day of the week. It also has a special instructional version that teaches students how to do the routine.

1. If the students have not done this week's routine before, play the instructional routine. If the PE teacher has already taught the routine to the students, or if they have already practiced the instructional routine with you, you can skip this step.
2. Play the Day 5 routine.

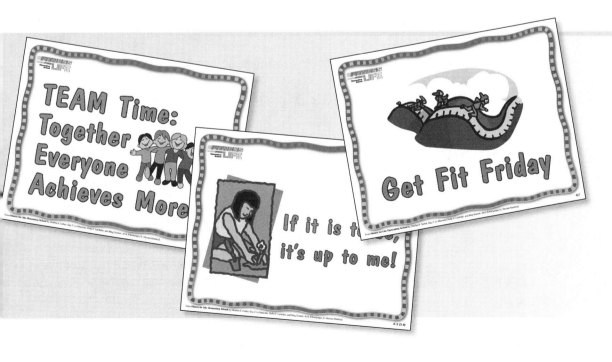

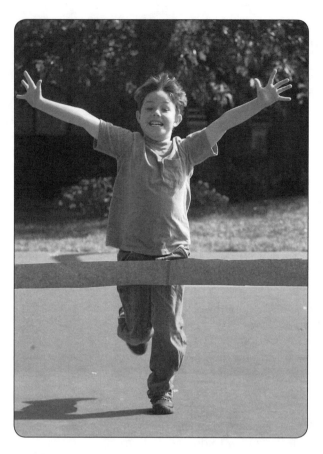

Trying hard and having a positive attitude lead to success.

Each day the current version of the routine promotes a new and different message. Variations on the message play before the first routine, between routines, and after the last routine. For Wave It, the Day 5 message is "If it is to be, it's up to me," and the three variations are as follows:

* Trying hard gets things done; trying hard makes you number one.

* It may be hard the first time I try, but with a few more tries, I can reach the sky. The choice is mine; it's up to me. I'll try real hard—watch and see.

* If I think I can, I can. If I think I can't, I can't. Whatever I think is right. I need to believe with all my might. You are in charge of how hard you will try, how you feel, and how you treat others.

## Breathing

After finishing the routine, lead the class in breathing.

"Breathing deeply is important for our bodies, so we'll end every activity with a couple of deep breaths. Let's all breathe in deeply (count 1, 2), hold (count 1, 2), breathe out (count 1, 2), and hold (count 1, 2)." Repeat three times.

## Background Information

* You can do so much if you believe in yourself!

* You are the boss of how hard you try.

* Talking to yourself and reminding yourself to keep trying is called positive self-talk. It really works.

* It is easier to keep trying if people around you encourage you. You can encourage people around you.

* When you believe you can do something, you can achieve!

## Discussion

* "Do you remember a time when you felt proud because you kept working at something that was hard?"

* "Show me what it looks like when you feel proud. That's right—people sit or stand up straight when they feel proud."

* "Can you think of some words to say to yourself or to someone else that would help you or him keep trying when things are hard?"

**teacher tip • • •**

"Nice time" refers to taking a few minutes to allow and encourage students to compliment each other on their work. Starting with a stem such as "I'd like to compliment _____ because she did a great job of _____" teaches the students how to identify a particular action to compliment. If you honor this time, the students will, too.

## Chant

Chanting is a great way to reinforce messages. If you've posted the corresponding sign, point to it, and tell the students that when you say the first phrase, they should respond by saying the second phrase. Make it fun!

> Teacher: "If it is to be . . ."
>
> Students: ". . . it's up to me!"

Practice several times until the students respond easily to your prompt.

## Closure

Closure provides an opportunity to focus one more time on the main message of the lesson by using compliments, reviewing messages, and making suggestions for doing activity at home. Closure also includes a brief preview of what's coming in the next lesson to help students see connections and begin to prepare for future lessons.

### *Compliments*

"You're getting so good at the routine that you can almost do it without thinking about it. As a class we are looking good!"

### *Take It Home*

* "Have you asked for more milk instead of soda at home?"
* "Have you eaten any dark green leafy vegetables? Which ones?"

> 🔄 **review** • • •
>
> "What does it feel like when people encourage you to keep trying? Think about the feelings you have when you keep trying and finally accomplish something you didn't think you could do. This week we did the Wave It routine. We've been talking about eating the right foods and exercising to get stronger."

* "Did you bring a healthy, protein-rich snack to school each day this week? What snacks did you bring?"
* "Are you still eating your 5 to 9 fruits and veggies a day?"
* "Have you gone for a walk or played with someone at home after school?"

### *Preview*

"During the next Wellness Week, we'll talk about energy."

# AFTERNOON ACTIVITY BREAK

**Activity**: Shoe Color Lineup

Perform in the afternoon or at some other time during the day when the students need a physical activity break.

"Remember, last Wellness Week we lined up in shirt color order. Today, we're going to line up in shoe color order. We'll use the rainbow for any colors and then go from darkest to lightest. So if your shoes are a color, listen for me to say that color. If your shoes are black, gray, brown, tan, or white, we'll go from darkest to lightest. If

> 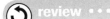 **interdisciplinary** • • •
>
> This activity requires practice in sequencing as well as movement.

your shoes have more than one color, go by whatever color shows the most. Here's a rainbow." (Show a picture of a rainbow—Roy G. Biv is an easy way to remember the order of the colors: red, orange, yellow, green, blue, indigo, and violet.) "When I say the color of your shoes, come get in line. We'll start with reds right here and make the line go that way. Ready? Red—all the reds come line up. Next, orange, yellow, green, blue, indigo, and violet. Let's put black, gray, brown, tan, and white at the end. Now, clap once, jump two times, march three times, and run in place four times. Now let's repeat that pattern."

Reinforce vocabulary about the relative position and magnitude of ordinal and cardinal numbers. You can use number operations when telling the students the number of times to do something (e.g., instead of telling them four times, use two plus two). Have students use addition, subtraction, less than, more than, and so on to determine the number of times to do each exercise.

## Breathing

After finishing the activity, lead the class in breathing.

"Breathing deeply is important for our bodies, so we'll end every activity with a couple of deep breaths. Let's all breathe in deeply (count 1, 2), hold (count 1, 2), breathe out (count 1, 2), and hold (count 1, 2)." Repeat three times.

## Closure

"You are good listeners and thinkers. Thanks for showing such good body control. On Wednesday you listened carefully when we played Simon Says. Yesterday you watched carefully when we played Follow the Leader. Today you worked as a team when we lined up by shoe color. I heard people helping each other figure out where they belonged by giving suggestions. I heard other people say, 'OK,' 'Thanks,' and 'Right.'"

# ADDITIONAL ACTIVITIES

See appendix A for additional enriching and integrative outdoor activities. For more information, go to www.fitnessforlife.org.

# WELLNESS WEEK 4

## Fitness for Life Elementary School

## Week 4 Overview

Table 2.4 is a summary chart of the Wellness Week 4 activities for the second grade classroom. Pages 111 through 134 provide the daily lesson plans for each day of week 4.

- Week 4 physical activity theme: Integration (energy balance)
- Week 4 nutrition theme: Healthy foods help us move

## Week 4 NASPE Standards

Week 4 activities meet the National Association for Sport and Physical Education (NASPE) standards listed here. For full standards and specific performance indicators (e.g., 1A through 6G), see appendix B.

- Standard 1: Motor skills and movement patterns, 1A, 1B, 1C, 1E, 1F
- Standard 2: Movement concepts and principles, 2C, 2D

## Table 2.4 Summary of Wellness Week 4 Activities

| Activity | Day 1 Monday | Day 2 Tuesday | Day 3 Wednesday | Day 4 Thursday | Day 5 Friday |
|---|---|---|---|---|---|
| Morning Activity Break | Video routine performed every day of the week: It's the One | | | | |
| Daily Message | Get off your seat and move your feet. | Play lots, learn lots. | Healthy food helps us move. | Be water wise. | Plan to get better. |
| Afternoon Activity Break | Alphabet Song | Pattern Practice | Simon Says | Follow the Leader | Birthday Lineup |
| Eat Well Wednesday Classroom Discussion | — | — | Eat Fat Sparingly; Avoid Empty Calories | — | — |
| Schoolwide Events | — | — | Eat Well Wednesday: Fruit and Veggie Bar With Bottled Water in the Cafeteria | — | Get Fit Friday: TEAM Time 4: Mid Kids Lead |

- Standard 3: Participates in physical activity, 3A, 3B, 3C
- Standard 4: Achieves health-enhancing physical fitness, 4A, 4B, 4C, 4D, 4E, 4F
- Standard 5: Exhibits responsible behavior and respect for others, 5A, 5B, 5C, 5G, 5H
- Standard 6: Values physical activity for health and social interactions, 6A, 6B, 6C, 6E, 6G

## Week 4 Math Standards

For specific focal points see appendix B.

- Numbers and operations (counting with understanding, ordinal and cardinal numbers)
- Algebra (sort, classify, order, sequence, pattern, add, subtract)
- Data analysis and probability (represent data using concrete objects, pictures, and graphs)

## Week 4 Standards for Other Curriculum Areas

Standards for other academic areas, such as sciences and language arts, were considered in developing lessons. Appendix B includes the sources of these standards.

## Week 4 Resources

There are three types of printed resources for use in Wellness Week 4: signs, worksheets, and newsletters. Web-based resources are also provided.

### Signs

General signs (described in more detail on page 17) can be used during Wellness Week 4 and reused in subsequent Wellness Weeks. Other signs are specifically for use during Wellness Week 4.

 **General**

G1: Fitness for Life: Elementary School

G2: Wellness Week

G3: Physical Activity Pyramid for Kids

G4: MyPyramid for Kids

G5: Eat Well Wednesday

G6: TEAM Time: Together Everyone Achieves More

G7: Get Fit Friday

G8: Healthy mind, healthy body, healthy heart . . . let's start!

G9: ABCs of Physical Activity

G10: ABCs of Nutrition

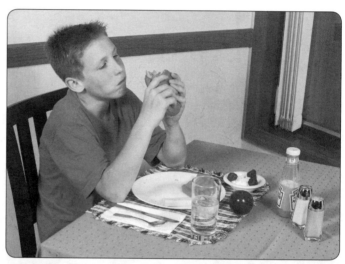

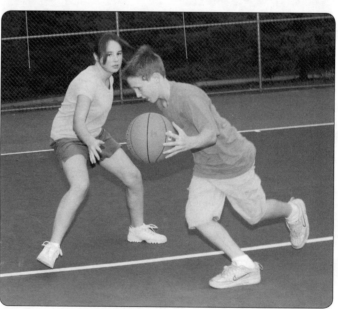

Lessons and messages in Wellness Week 4 emphasize the idea of integration or energy balance (balancing the energy taken in through food with the energy expended through activity).

**Wellness Week 4 → Signs**

4.1: Physical Activity Pyramid: Do activities from all the steps!

4.2: Eat all of the colors in the pyramid!

*4.3: Get off your seat and move your feet!

*4.4: Get up, get moving, and have some fun. It helps your brain when you get out and run!

4.5: Play lots, learn lots!

*4.6: Play every day, sun or rain. Playing is good for your brain!

4.7: Energy in (the food we eat) – energy out (how much we move) = a healthy body

*4.8: Healthy foods help us move! Choose your foods wisely!

4.9: Everyday foods versus sometimes foods

4.10: Be water wise!

4.11: Be sun wise!

*4.12: Sweating cools your body when you start to get hot. Take breaks and drink water if you want to play a lot.

*4.13: If you want to do better than before, make a plan to practice more!

4.14: Make a plan to get fit. Set a goal and go for it!

---

\* Indicates signs used for chants

## Worksheets

The DVD includes black-and-white versions of all Week 4 signs that you can print and use as coloring worksheets. In addition, the DVD includes black-and-white versions of MyPyramid for Kids and the Physical Activity Pyramid for Kids for coloring.

 **Wellness Week 4 → Worksheets**

## Newsletters

The DVD contains a newsletter for use during each Wellness Week. It is recommended that

 **teacher tip • • •**

Choose a bulletin board to use for wellness in your classroom. During each Wellness Week, post the general signs all week. Each day of Wellness Week, feature the signs of the day or post all daily signs and point out the sign of the day on appropriate days. If possible, feature the sign of the day at the front of the classroom. At the end of Wellness Week, continue to feature wellness on the wellness bulletin board, rotating signs from time to time.

your wellness coordinator edit, print, and distribute these newsletters. If you do not have a wellness coordinator, or if your coordinator does not handle the newsletters, you can do it yourself. Just open the appropriate newsletter file, follow the instructions to edit and customize the newsletter, print it, and distribute it, either electronically or by sending copies home with the students. Remind students to talk to their families about Wellness Week and the information in the newsletters.

 **Wellness Week 4 → Newsletter**

## Web Resources

Available at www.mypyramid.gov: a My-Pyramid worksheet and nutrition activities

Available at www.dole.com/superkids/: *Kids Cookbook*, games, puzzles, and other nutrition activities

# Week 4 Special Days

Each Wellness Week, two schoolwide activities are featured. On Eat Well Wednesday, nutrition is the focus, and on Get Fit Friday, physical activity is the focus. These activities provide opportunities for the whole school to have a common experience and to highlight the importance of nutrition and physical activity to health and wellness.

## Eat Well Wednesday

During each Wellness Week, Day 3 (typically Wednesday) is known as Eat Well Wednesday. On this day, teachers and staff are encouraged to emphasize the weekly nutrition message. Special schoolwide events (e.g., a lunch salad bar or healthy snack preparation) may be planned by the wellness coordinator. Teachers are encouraged to support these Eat Well Wednesday events and plan special Eat Well Wednesday events in their classrooms, emphasizing sound nutrition. During Wellness Week 4, a special fruit, vegetable, and water bar will be set up in the cafeteria.

### Get Fit Friday

During each Wellness Week, Day 5 (typically Friday) is known as Get Fit Friday. On this day, a schoolwide event focusing on physical activity will be planned by the wellness coordinator. The Get Fit Friday activities are called TEAM Time activities (TEAM stands for Together Everyone Achieves More).

During Wellness Week 4, the TEAM Time activity planned for Get Fit Friday is called Mid Kids Lead. The wellness coordinator will teach several third and fourth grade students how to do the routine ahead of time so that they can help lead. Then the wellness coordinator and the selected students will lead the TEAM Time activity at the beginning of the school day. All students in the school will congregate outside or in the gym or multipurpose room so that they all can participate together. The activity includes a warm-up, a workout routine, and a cool-down.

### ACES Day

May is National Physical Fitness Month and the first week in May is National Physical Education Week. In 1984 Len Saunders created a program called Project ACES (All Children Exercising Simultaneously). Each year in the first week of May, children throughout the world participate in Project ACES by doing exercises at the same time on the same day. The children in your school can participate by performing the TEAM Time activity on ACES Day at the designated time. More information is available at http://lensaunders.com/aces/aces.html.

# USING THE VIDEO ACTIVITIES

During each Wellness Week, you will play an activity video every day. The five videos use the same activity routine but present different conceptual messages for each day of the week. Simply play the appropriate video and have your students perform the routine for that day. The DVD also provides an instructional video for each week's routine. If your school has a physical education teacher, he or she may have taught the routine to students during the week before Wellness Week, in which case you won't have to use the instructional video. Otherwise, you can use it to help your students learn the routine.

In the instructional video, the instructor faces away from your students for some of the left–right movements. Explain to students that they should do those movements the same way the instructor does them. That is, when the instructor moves to the right, they should also move to the right. However, in the daily activity videos, the leaders face forward, so their left–right movements are in reverse (mirror image). While following along with the daily activity videos, your students should move in the opposite direction of the leaders for left–right movements. Keep in mind that although moving in the correct direction is desirable, the key is to get all kids moving regardless of the direction. If your students have a hard time performing the activity, feel free to replay the instructional video.

# WELLNESS WEEK 4

## Day 1 Lesson Plan

## OVERVIEW

* **Morning Activity Break**: It's the One (DVD routine)
* **Afternoon Activity Break**: Alphabet Song

## OBJECTIVES

Students will

* participate in 10 minutes of moderate to vigorous physical activity;
* repeat the message that physical activity is good for their brains; and
* participate in physical activity, making only supportive comments to themselves and others.

## RESOURCES

### Signs

 **General**

G2: Wellness Week

G3: Physical Activity Pyramid for Kids

G8: Healthy mind, healthy body, healthy heart . . . let's start!

 **Wellness Week 4 → Signs**

4.1: Physical Activity Pyramid: Do activities from all the steps!

4.2: Eat all of the colors in the pyramid!

* 4.3: Get off your seat and move your feet!

* 4.4: Get up, get moving, and have some fun. It helps your brain when you get out and run!

---

* Indicates signs used for chants

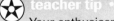 **teacher tip • • •**
Your enthusiasm will go a long way to "sell" physical activity as an important part of daily life. Focus on enjoying this active time yourself as well as on the importance of it for your children's minds and bodies!

### Worksheets

The DVD includes black-and-white versions of today's signs that you can print and use as coloring worksheets. In addition, the DVD includes black-and-white versions of MyPyramid for Kids and the Physical Activity Pyramid for Kids for coloring.

 **Wellness Week 4 → Worksheets**

# MORNING ACTIVITY BREAK

**DVD Routine**: It's the One

## Introduction

"Being physically active every day is important not just for our bodies but also for our brains. We think best when we are alert. We are more alert when we exercise. This week we're going to be talking about balancing the energy we take into our bodies by eating with the energy we use when we are active. Let's watch this video and use some of our energy."

> **? comprehension check • • •**
>
> "Point to your movement space. That's right, move in just one place, not around the room."
>
> "Before we start, let's go over a special signal. When I clap my hands like this"—clap your hands three times, or choose your own attention signal—"I want you to stop moving and look at me. Let's practice. Start marching in place. (Clap, clap, clap.) Great job stopping and looking right at me!"

## Video Routine

The DVD has five versions of the It's the One routine, one for each day of the week. It also has a special instructional version that teaches students how to do the routine.

1. Play the instructional routine. If the PE teacher has already taught the routine to the students, you can skip this step.
2. Play the Day 1 routine.

Each day the current version of the routine promotes a new and different message. Variations on the message play before the first routine, between routines, and after

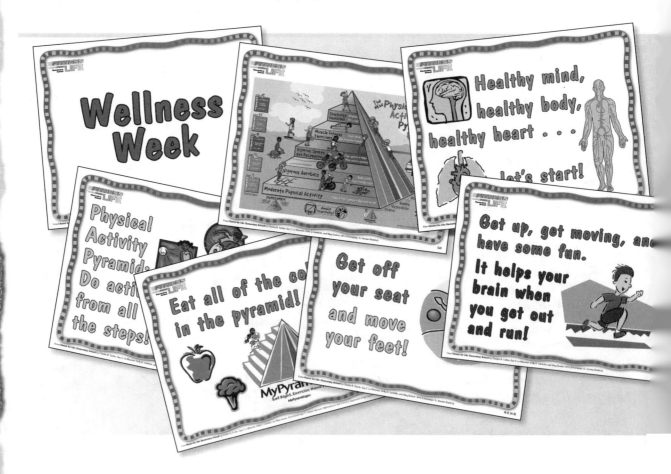

WEEK **4** • DAY **1**

the last routine. For It's the One, the Day 1 message is "Get off your seat and move your feet," and the three variations are as follows:

* Your brain gets working when you get on your feet; moving your body is a special treat.

* Too much sitting makes you a couch potato; get up and move like a swirling tornado.

* When you move around, you need your many senses like sight, sound, balance, and touch. Watching TV uses only sight and sound. Get out, get moving, and have some fun—you do your brain good when you get out and run.

> 👁 **observation** • • •
> Look around the room. Are the children showing good body control? If anyone is, praise him; if not, restate your expectations.

## Breathing

After finishing the routine, lead the class in breathing.

"Breathing deeply is important for our bodies, so we'll end every activity with a couple of deep breaths. Let's all breathe in deeply (count 1, 2), hold (count 1, 2), breathe out (count 1, 2), and hold (count 1, 2)." Repeat three times.

## Background Information

* Movement and activity have been linked to better cognitive functioning.

* When you move around, your heart beats faster and pumps your blood to all parts of your body. Blood carries oxygen and so gives your brain more oxygen.

* When you are active, your brain makes special chemicals that help you feel good and help the brain make connections between brain cells.

* To maintain a healthy weight, move more and sit less!

## Discussion

* Point to the Physical Activity Pyramid for Kids. Emphasize the need for different kinds of activity.

* "How much time to you think you spend watching TV each day?"

* "How much time to you spend in active play?"

* "What are some good activities you could do instead of watching TV?"

* "Do you feel more alert after you have been active?"

## Chant

Chanting is a great way to reinforce messages. If you've posted the corresponding sign, point to it, and tell the students that when you say the first phrase, they should respond by saying the second phrase. Make it fun!

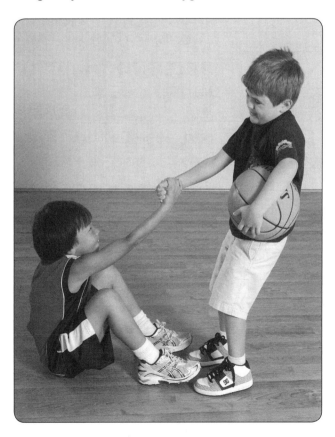

Get off your seat and move your feet! Activity is good for your body and your brain.

Teacher: "Get off your seat . . ."

Students: ". . . and move your feet!"

Teacher: "Get up, get moving, and have some fun."

Students: "It helps your brain when you get out and run!"

Practice several times until the students respond easily to your prompt.

## Closure

Closure provides an opportunity to focus one more time on the main message of the lesson by using compliments, reviewing messages, and making suggestions for doing activity at home. Closure also includes a brief preview of what's coming in the next lesson to help students see connections and begin to prepare for future lessons.

> **review** • • •
> "Do you feel more alert after you are active? Today we talked about how being active helps our brain and how being active takes energy. We get energy from food and use it to be active."

### Compliments

"You did a great job moving and following the video. You used a lot of energy."

### Take It Home

"Name one physical activity you will do at home today."

### Preview

"Since this is Wellness Week, we're really going to try to be especially active. We're going to take a break like this every day and move."

# AFTERNOON ACTIVITY BREAK

**Activity**: Alphabet Song

Perform in the afternoon or at some other time during the day when the students need a physical activity break.

> **interdisciplinary** • • •
> This activity incorporates the letters of the alphabet while students are moving.

Sing the alphabet song while marching in place. Have the students make the shapes of the easy letters (A, C, I, M, T, X, Y) with their bodies. (Have them practice first.)

Consider using the following extensions:

* Have the children raise their hands when they sing the first letter of their first name, the first letter of their last name, or any letters in their name.
* Change the locomotor pattern (e.g., hop, skip, gallop, or walk).
* Have students try singing the alphabet song backward for a challenge.

## Breathing

After finishing the activity, lead the class in breathing.

"Breathing deeply is important for our bodies, so we'll end every activity with a couple of deep breaths. Let's all breathe in deeply (count 1, 2), hold (count 1, 2), breathe out (count 1, 2), and hold (count 1, 2)." Repeat three times.

WEEK 4 • DAY 1

## Closure

"Thanks for showing such good body control. You all did that without any problems even though we are in a small space. Since you have such good body control, we'll be able to do lots of fun things because I won't have to worry about you getting hurt when you are moving in this little space."

# ADDITIONAL ACTIVITIES

See appendix A for additional enriching and integrative outdoor activities. For more information, go to www.fitnessforlife.org.

## Day 2 Lesson Plan ● ● ● ● ● ● ● ● ● ● ● ● ● ● ● ● ● ● ●

### OVERVIEW

* **Morning Activity Break**: It's the One (DVD routine)
* **Afternoon Activity Break**: Pattern Practice

### OBJECTIVES

Students will

* participate in 10 minutes of moderate to vigorous physical activity;
* repeat the message that music helps everyone enjoy moving;
* participate in physical activity, making only supportive comments to themselves and others; and
* identify the correct movement to continue an ABCD pattern and perform the pattern of movements.

### RESOURCES

**Signs**

 **Wellness Week 4 → Signs**

4.5: Play lots, learn lots!

* 4.6: Play every day, sun or rain. Playing is good for your brain!

---

\* Indicates sign used for chant

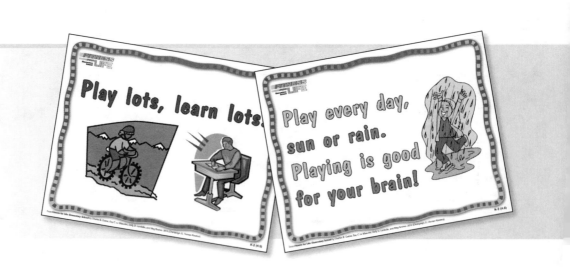

## Worksheets

The DVD includes black-and-white versions of today's signs that you can print and use as coloring worksheets. In addition, the DVD includes black-and-white versions of MyPyramid for Kids and the Physical Activity Pyramid for Kids for coloring.

 **Wellness Week 4 → Worksheets**

# MORNING ACTIVITY BREAK

**DVD Routine**: It's the One

## Introduction

"Yesterday we talked about how moving helps our brains. Playing and moving keeps us more alert, and being alert makes it easier to learn new things. This song helps you to get active."

## Video Routine

The DVD has five versions of the It's the One routine, one for each day of the week. It also has a special instructional version that teaches students how to do the routine.

1. If the students have not done this week's routine before, play the instructional routine. If the PE teacher has already taught the routine to the students, or if they have already practiced the instructional routine with you, you can skip this step.
2. Play the Day 2 routine.

Each day the current version of the routine promotes a new and different message. Variations on the message play before the first routine, between routines, and after the last routine. For It's the One, the Day 2 message is "Play lots, learn lots," and the three variations are as follows:

* When you play lots of games with family and friends, learning new skills will never end.
* The more activities that you do, the more you'll learn—yes, that means you!
* Trying lots of different physical activities helps us build many skills and meet many different people. The more you try, the more you'll know; the more you try, your friends will grow.

## Breathing

After finishing the routine, lead the class in breathing.

"Breathing deeply is important for our bodies, so we'll end every activity with a couple of deep breaths. Let's all breathe in deeply (count 1, 2), hold (count 1, 2), breathe out (count 1, 2), and hold (count 1, 2)." Repeat three times.

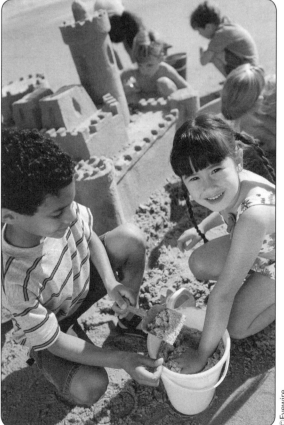

©Eyewire

Children can learn new skills and make friends by trying many different activities and games.

## Background Information

* The more different physical activities you try, the better chance you have of meeting new friends.

* If you learn new skills and activities, you have more ways to be active.

* When you play, your imagination gets practice, and you learn to think creatively.

* You learn lots about the world when playing—like gravity pulls things (including us) toward the earth. If we jump up, we must come down.

## Discussion

* "What are some of your favorite activities to do at recess?"

* "What kinds of skills would you like to learn?" (Answers might include jump rope, catch, or tap dance.)

* "Do you remember any special things you have learned while playing?"

> **teacher tip** • • •
> Chanting can be fun and really help remind us of important points. Be enthusiastic, use different accents, and allow the students to shout back their responses sometimes. Encourage students to teach the chants to their families.

## Chant

Chanting is a great way to reinforce messages. If you've posted the corresponding sign, point to it, and tell the students that when you say the first phrase, they should respond by saying the second phrase. Make it fun!

Teacher: "Play every day . . ."

Students: ". . . sun or rain!"

Teacher: "Playing is good . . ."

Students: ". . . for your brain!"

Practice several times until the students respond easily to your prompt.

## Closure

Closure provides an opportunity to focus one more time on the main message of the lesson by using compliments, reviewing messages, and making suggestions for doing activity at home. Closure also includes a brief preview of what's coming in the next lesson to help students see connections and begin to prepare for future lessons.

### Compliments

"You did a great job following the video. There were lots of movements to do in the song—stepping, sliding, and jumping. You were listening, and you're getting better and better. Moving is good for your body!"

### Take It Home

"Combine a skill you learned in PE with a skill you learned in the classroom, like jumping rope while spelling or skipping while counting."

> **review** • • •
> "Think about a time when you noticed something new when you were playing—maybe a flower, the wind in your face, or a footprint in the dirt. Today we talked about learning new things when you are playing."

### Preview

"Tomorrow we'll talk about getting energy from the foods we eat."

WEEK 4 • DAY 2

# AFTERNOON ACTIVITY BREAK

**Activity**: Pattern Practice

Perform in the afternoon or at some other time when the students need a physical activity break.

"Do you remember that when we did our lineup activity, we did some movements? Let's do it by our desks. Clap once, jump two times, march three times, and run four times. This is a new kind of pattern. We do the first thing one time, the second thing two times, the third thing three times, and the fourth thing four times. If we were to add one more movement to our pattern, like waving, how many times do you think we would do it? Right! Five times because we did the first thing one time, the second thing two times, the third thing three times, and the fourth thing four times, so now we would do the fifth thing five times." Add things to do six, seven, eight, nine and 10 times to your sequence.

> **interdisciplinary • • •**
> This activity helps students practice patterns in movement. Being able to recognize, follow, and create patterns are also important skills in math.

You can also use number operations when telling the students the number of times to do something (e.g., instead of telling them four times, use two plus two). Have students use addition, subtraction, less than, more than, and so on to determine the number of times to do each exercise.

## Breathing

After finishing the activity, lead the class in breathing.

"Breathing deeply is important for our bodies, so we'll end every activity with a couple of deep breaths. Let's all breathe in deeply (count 1, 2), hold (count 1, 2), breathe out (count 1, 2), and hold (count 1, 2)." Repeat three times.

## Closure

"Wow! You're great at patterns. We can make up lots of patterns to do. It just takes practice to get good at them. Thanks for showing such good body control. You all did that without any problems even though we are in a small space. Since you have such good body control, we can keep doing active games in the classroom. I won't have to worry about you getting hurt when you are moving in this little space."

# ADDITIONAL ACTIVITIES

See appendix A for additional enriching and integrative outdoor activities. For more information, go to www.fitnessforlife.org.

WEEK **4** • DAY **2**

# 4 WELLNESS WEEK

## Day 3 Lesson Plan

### OVERVIEW

* **Morning Activity Break**: It's the One (DVD routine)
* **Eat Well Wednesday Class Discussion**: Eat Fat Sparingly; Avoid Empty Calories
* **Eat Well Wednesday Activity**: Fruit and Veggie Bar With Bottled Water in the Cafeteria
* **Afternoon Activity Break**: Simon Says

### OBJECTIVES

Students will

* participate in 10 minutes of moderate to vigorous physical activity,
* repeat (correctly) the message that healthy food helps them move,
* practice decision making and attention by responding with movement on appropriate verbal cues (Simon Says) and not responding when the cue is missing,
* identify the color stripe on the food pyramid associated with oils (or fat, in yellow), and
* describe energy balance (the energy that goes into your body should equal the energy used by your body).

### RESOURCES

#### Signs

 **General**

G4: MyPyramid for Kids

G5: Eat Well Wednesday

G10: ABCs of Nutrition

 **Wellness Week 4 → Signs**

4.7: Energy in (the food we eat) – energy out (how much we move) = a healthy body

\* 4.8: Healthy foods help us move! Choose your foods wisely!

4.9: Everyday foods versus sometimes foods

———————

\* Indicates sign used for chant

## Worksheets

The DVD includes black-and-white versions of today's signs that you can print and use as coloring worksheets. In addition, the DVD includes black-and-white versions of MyPyramid for Kids and the Physical Activity Pyramid for Kids for coloring.

 **Wellness Week 4 → Worksheets**

## Web Resources

Additional activities available at www.mypyramid.gov and www.dole.com/superkids/.

# MORNING ACTIVITY BREAK

**DVD Routine**: It's the One

## Introduction

"Wellness Week reminds us of things we should be doing every week and every day. Yesterday we talked about learning through playing. Today we'll talk about how foods give us energy. If you don't use the energy in the food you eat, it gets stored in your body as fat. Using energy is good for your body. Doing the routine today should be easier today because this is our third day trying it. Show me your good body control again today."

## Video Routine

The DVD has five versions of the It's the One routine, one for each day of the week. It also has a special instructional version that teaches students how to do the routine.

1. If the students have not done this week's routine before, play the instructional routine. If the PE teacher has already taught the routine to the students, or if they have already practiced the instructional routine with you, you can skip this step.

2. Play the Day 3 routine.

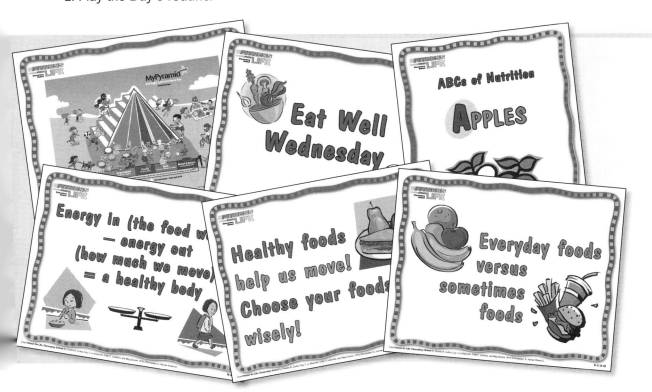

WEEK 4 • DAY 3

**observation • • •**

Look around the room. Are the children showing good body control? Are there any parts of the routine that are particularly hard, creating stumbling blocks for the students? Note any so you can either have the students practice that piece or modify the routine to allow them to flow through it.

Each day the current version of the routine promotes a new and different message. Variations on the message play before the first routine, between routines, and after the last routine. For It's the One, the Day 3 message is "Healthy food helps us move," and the three variations are as follows:

* Did you know that the food you eat gives you energy to move your feet?

* Eat healthy food for breakfast, lunch, and dinner. Eating healthy food can make us winners.

* The food we eat gives us energy to ride our bikes, dance, and play hide and seek. Healthy food like fruits and vegetables gives us the energy we need and gives us vitamins to grow healthy.

## Breathing

After finishing the routine, lead the class in breathing.

"Breathing deeply is important for our bodies, so we'll end every activity with a couple of deep breaths. Let's all breathe in deeply (count 1, 2), hold (count 1, 2), breathe out (count 1, 2), and hold (count 1, 2)." Repeat three times.

## Background Information

* Calories are the measure of how much energy is in our food.

* Some foods provide calories that are converted to energy more easily than others.

* Fruits and vegetables are carbohydrates that give us good energy.

* Vitamins help keep our cells working well but don't have calories.

* Healthy food helps us move.

## Discussion

* "Have you ever tried to run around after eating a big meal? What does it feel like?"

* "The gas we put in the car gives it energy to make the engine turn the wheels. The food we put in our bodies give us the energy to move our muscles. Fruits and vegetables give us good energy. Right after we exercise, chocolate skim milk helps our cells rebuild."

* "What fruits and veggies do you like to eat to give you energy?"

## Chant

Chanting is a great way to reinforce messages. If you've posted the corresponding sign,

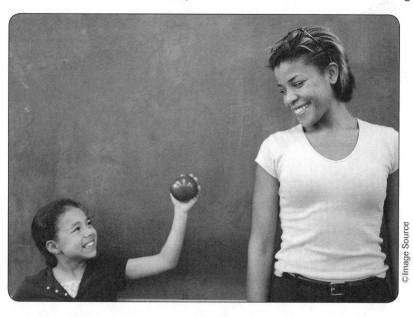

©Image Source

Healthy foods like fruits provide energy for movement and vitamins for healthy growth.

point to it, and tell the students that when you say the first phrase, they should respond by saying the second phrase. Make it fun!

Teacher: "Healthy foods . . ."

Students: ". . . help us move!"

Teacher: "Choose your foods . . ."

Students: ". . . wisely!"

Practice several times until the students respond easily to your prompt.

## Closure

Closure provides an opportunity to focus one more time on the main message of the lesson by using compliments, reviewing messages, and making suggestions for doing activity at home. Closure also includes a brief preview of what's coming in the next lesson to help students see connections and begin to prepare for future lessons.

### Compliments

"You did lots of good exercising while singing It's the One. I saw lots of great energy being used."

### Take It Home

**↺ review • • •**

"Today we talked about eating good foods and exercising to balance our energy. Think of yourself as a car. Eating food is like filling up at the gas station. You can't fill it up again until you have driven and used up some of the gas."

"After you have been playing hard is a good time for a glass of chocolate milk. Try it sometime. Make your own with skim milk and chocolate syrup. It has protein and carbohydrates, and right after a lot of exercise, it helps your muscles get stronger."

### Preview

"Tomorrow we're going to be talking about the importance of drinking water."

# EAT WELL WEDNESDAY

Each Wednesday all teachers and staff are encouraged to emphasize the weekly nutrition message. Special schoolwide events (e.g., a lunch salad bar or healthy snack preparation) may be planned by the wellness coordinator. Teachers are encouraged to support these Eat Well Wednesday events and plan special Eat Well Wednesday events in their classrooms, emphasizing sound nutrition.

## Eat Well Wednesday Class Discussion

**Nutrition Topic**: Eat Fat Sparingly; Avoid Empty Calories

### Introduction

The main theme is balancing calories. You should take in the same number of calories in your diet that you use in physical activity. Eat from all food groups. MyPyramid provides guidelines for healthy eating and introduces the five food groups: grains, vegetables, fruits, milk, and meat and beans. Oils (not a food group) are also pictured in MyPyramid to aid the discussion of fat: which types are good and which are not so good.

### Background Information

* When you treat your body well, it will grow, keep itself strong, and heal itself when hurt.
* Nutrients are elements in healthy foods with special jobs. There are six nutrient types (carbohydrate, vitamins, minerals, fat, protein, and water).

* By eating a wide variety of foods, every color every day, your body receives all the nutrients it needs to learn, move, and grow.

* Your body uses energy found in food. Energy is measured in calories. If you eat more calories than your body needs, your body stores the extra energy as fat. Your body needs some fat for energy, protection, and warmth.

* There are healthy kinds of fat and some not-so-healthy kinds of fat. Fat is found in many foods like bacon, muffins, cheese, and ice cream. Fatty foods lead to low energy and poor work at school.

* Foods with lots of sugar give us an energy burst, but they generally have little nutritional value, and the energy burst doesn't last very long. Also, if we don't burn all the calories through activity, those foods add extra weight to our bodies.

* Fruits do not contain fat and extra sugar and are a good source of energy.

### Discussion

* "How can we tell what kind of fat is in our food or how many calories are in our foods?"

* Have some snack containers available so you can look at the nutrition label to determine the calories and fat in the different snacks. (For instance, compare the number of fat calories in a box of Wheat Thins with those in a bag of Sun Chips. Or compare Goldfish with raisins.)

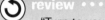 review • • •

• "Turn to your neighbor and name three different foods that do not contain fat." (Examples include fruits and veggies.)

• "Name one way you can reduce the amount of fat in a favorite food." (For example, you could use low-fat milk rather than whole milk, or choose low-fat ice cream.)

### Take It Home

* "Find out a family member's favorite high-energy snack. How many fat calories does it have?"

* "Plan, with your family, a healthy snack like an apple (low in fat grams) for after school each day."

* "Go shopping with your family and look at the food labels when buying energy-rich snack choices. Less than a third of the calories in energy-rich foods should come from fat."

### Eat Well Wednesday Schoolwide Activity

During Wellness Week 4, a special fruit, vegetable, and water bar will be set up in the cafeteria.

## AFTERNOON ACTIVITY BREAK

**Activity**: Simon Says

Perform in the afternoon or at some other time during the day when the students need a physical activity break.

interdisciplinary • • •

This activity includes movement and helps students practice categorizing skills since they have to put the instructions into one of two categories: instructions to follow and instructions to ignore. The activity also provides practice in number operations by using various methods for defining the number of times to do each movement.

Begin by explaining how the game works. Tell them that when you start an instruction with "Simon says," they should do what you say. But if you simply tell them to do something, such as "Wave your arms," they shouldn't

WEEK 4 • DAY 3

respond. Then lead them through several examples so they understand how the game works. For instance, if you say, "Simon says, 'Put your hands on your hips,'" the students should put their hands on their hips. But if you say, "Jump up and down three times," they should just stay still since you didn't say "Simon says". If the students mess up, don't worry, just go on to the next action.

You can use number operations when telling the students the number of times to do something (e.g., instead of saying four, use two plus two). Have students use addition, subtraction, less than, more than, and so on to determine the number of times to do each exercise. Reinforce the vocabulary about the relative position and magnitude of ordinal and cardinal numbers when talking about their position in the line and related situations.

> **? comprehension check** • • •
> "Show me what you will do if I say, 'Simon says, "Touch your shoulders."'" Show me what you will do if I say, 'Touch your knees' without saying, 'Simon says.'"

If students make mistakes just say, "Oops," laugh with them, and then go on with the next action. Do lots of fun movements. End up with more gentle movements so they calm down slowly, and the heart slows down gradually.

## Breathing

After finishing the activity, lead the class in breathing.

"Breathing deeply is important for our bodies, so we'll end every activity with a couple of deep breaths. Let's all breathe in deeply (count 1, 2), hold (count 1, 2), breathe out (count 1, 2), and hold (count 1, 2)." Repeat three times.

## Closure

"Thanks for showing such good body control. You paid careful attention to what Simon said to do. That's careful listening. Careful listening helps you learn lots of new things. You also helped burn up some of the energy from the food you ate for lunch."

> **★ teacher tip** • • •
> Try to make discussions about foods empowering for children. Focus on the foods that will help build their bodies and celebrate the enjoyment and empowerment associated with choosing nutritious foods.

# ADDITIONAL ACTIVITIES

See appendix A for additional enriching and integrative outdoor activities. For more information, go to www.fitnessforlife.org.

## Day **4** Lesson Plan ·············

### OVERVIEW

✳ **Morning Activity Break**: It's the One (DVD routine)

✳ **Afternoon Activity Break**: Follow the Leader

### OBJECTIVES

Students will

✳ participate in 10 minutes of moderate to vigorous physical activity;

✳ repeat the message that doing a little more even when they are tired helps their muscles get stronger;

✳ participate in physical activity, making only supportive comments to themselves and others; and

✳ count movements appropriately.

### RESOURCES

**Signs**

 **Wellness Week 4 → Signs**

4.10: Be water wise!

4.11: Be sun wise!

\* 4.12: Sweating cools your body when you start to get hot. Take breaks and drink water if you want to play a lot.

_____
\* Indicates sign used for chant

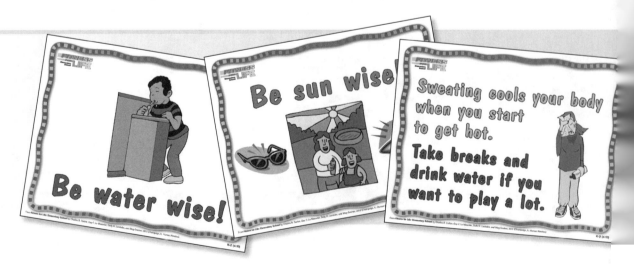

## Worksheets

The DVD includes black-and-white versions of today's signs that you can print and use as coloring worksheets. In addition, the DVD includes black-and-white versions of MyPyramid for Kids and the Physical Activity Pyramid for Kids for coloring.

 **Wellness Week 4 → Worksheets**

# MORNING ACTIVITY BREAK

**DVD Routine**: It's the One

## Introduction

"Yesterday we talked about how healthy food gives us energy to move. Water helps your body cool itself and helps all the cells in your body work right. Drinking eight glasses of water every day is good for you."

## Video Routine

The DVD has five versions of the It's the One routine, one for each day of the week. It also has a special instructional version that teaches students how to do the routine.

1. If the students have not done this week's routine before, play the instructional routine. If the PE teacher has already taught the routine to the students, or if they have already practiced the instructional routine with you, you can skip this step.
2. Play the Day 4 routine.

Each day the current version of the routine promotes a new and different message. Variations on the message play before the first routine, between routines, and after the last routine. For It's the One, the Day 4 message is "Be water wise," and the three variations are as follows:

* Your body loses water when you sweat. Drinking lots of water is the best plan yet.
* Sweating cools your body when you start to get hot. Take breaks and drink water if you want to play a lot.
* Your body needs water to keep your insides cool; taking lots of drinks when playing is a pretty good rule.

## Breathing

After finishing the routine, lead the class in breathing.

> 👁 **observation** • • •
> Look around the room. Are the students doing the activity with ease? Tell them how well they are doing and how much better they have gotten with practice.

"Breathing deeply is important for our bodies, so we'll end every activity with a couple of deep breaths. Let's all breathe in deeply (count 1, 2), hold (count 1, 2), breathe out (count 1, 2), and hold (count 1, 2)." Repeat three times.

## Background Information

* Water is an essential nutrient that helps the body regulate its temperature through sweating.
* Plain water is the best drink you can take when being active.
* Drinking eight glasses of water a day is good for your body.

WEEK 4 • DAY 4

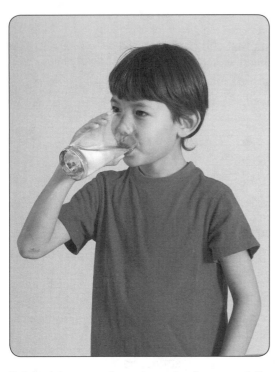

Drink plain water throughout the day, especially when engaging in physical activity.

* When it is hot out or you are moving a lot, you lose water by sweating, and you need to drink even more.
* More than half of your body is water!

## Discussion

* "When is it OK for you to get a drink of water in this class?"
* "Where else can you get drinks of water?" (Answers might include at the playground, at home, or in the lunchroom.)
* "What helps you remember to drink water every day?"

## Chant

Chanting is a great way to reinforce messages. If you've posted the corresponding sign, point to it, and tell the students that when you say the first phrase, they should respond by saying the second phrase. Make it fun!

Teacher: "Sweating cools your body when you start to get hot."

Students: "Take breaks and drink water if you want to play a lot!"

Practice several times until the students respond easily to your prompt.

## Closure

Closure provides an opportunity to focus one more time on the main message of the lesson by using compliments, reviewing messages, and making suggestions for doing activity at home. Closure also includes a brief preview of what's coming in the next lesson to help students see connections and begin to prepare for future lessons.

### *Compliments*

"You're getting so good at the routine that it looks like you can almost do it without thinking about it. You are getting good enough to sing along as you are doing it. It's hard to do that when you are first learning the routine. When you exercise like that, you need to remember to drink more water."

### *Take It Home*

"Can you think of ways to remember to drink water at home? How about having a glass of water when you brush your teeth or eat a meal? Drink water at home in the morning before school, at home after school, and before or after you play."

🔄 **review** • • •
"You need to drink water every day and more when you exercise. Think about the cues that remind you to drink water, like seeing the water fountain or getting up in the morning. Don't wait until you are really thirsty before getting a drink."

### *Preview*

"This week we talked about balancing the food we eat and the energy we use. Tomorrow we'll talk about how to make a good plan if we need to do something different from what we have been doing."

WEEK 4 • DAY 4

# AFTERNOON ACTIVITY BREAK

**Activity**: Follow the Leader

Perform in the afternoon or at some other time during the day when the students need a physical activity break.

**teacher tip** • • •
Sharing positive expectations and what helpful behavior looks like and sounds like can go a long way to helping children enjoy participation in movement settings. For example, you might say: "Sometimes things are hard to do. What could a person do to get back on track if she made a mistake? What might you say to someone to encourage him to keep trying when he was getting tired?"

Begin by telling the students, "In Follow the Leader you do just what I do. Ready? Here we go." Start with simple actions; for example, put your hands in the air and wave them back and forth. Try to do at least 8 counts of each movement. So you might march in place and count 1, 2, 3, 4, 5, 6, 7, 8; clap your hands 1, 2, 3, 4, 5, 6, 7, 8; or run in place. Have fun with it. Add harder actions like jump rope skills without a rope (ski jumps, bell jumps, criss-crosses, single bounces, or double bounces). When you get near the end of the exercise, do slower movements to allow their hearts to slow down again. Tell them you are doing this. Keep counting from one movement to another, explaining that you are counting to 50 by doing 5 sets of 10 movements.

## Breathing

After finishing the activity, lead the class in breathing.

"Breathing deeply is important for our bodies, so we'll end every activity with a couple of deep breaths. Let's all breathe in deeply (count 1, 2), hold (count 1, 2), breathe out (count 1, 2), and hold (count 1, 2)." Repeat three times.

## Closure

"You worked hard today and used lots of energy. Yesterday you paid careful attention to what Simon said. Today you worked hard and paid careful attention to what I was doing. That's careful watching. Being able to watch carefully and copy what you see helps you learn lots of skills."

# ADDITIONAL ACTIVITIES

See appendix A for additional enriching and integrative outdoor activities. For more information, go to www.fitnessforlife.org.

WEEK 4 • DAY 4

# Day 5 Lesson Plan

## OVERVIEW

* **Get Fit Friday Activity:** TEAM Time 4: Mid Kids Lead
* **Morning Activity Break**: It's the One (DVD routine)
* **Afternoon Activity Break**: Birthday Lineup

## OBJECTIVES

Students will

* participate in 10 minutes of moderate to vigorous physical activity;
* move fluidly and confidently during the video routine;
* repeat the message that if they want to get better, it is good to write a plan;
* demonstrate understanding of a bar graph by identifying the most common birthday month;
* participate in physical activity, making only supportive comments to themselves and others; and
* be team members who try to help the team accomplish the task (Birthday Lineup).

## RESOURCES

### Signs

 **General**

G6: TEAM Time: Together Everyone Achieves More
G7: Get Fit Friday

 **Wellness Week 4 → Signs**

* 4.13: If you want to do better than before, make a plan to practice more!
 4.14: Make a plan to get fit. Set a goal and go for it!

---

* Indicates sign used for chant

### Worksheets

The DVD includes black-and-white versions of today's signs that you can print and use as coloring worksheets. In addition, the DVD includes black-and-white versions of MyPyramid for Kids and the Physical Activity Pyramid for Kids for coloring.

 **Wellness Week 4 → Worksheets**

## GET FIT FRIDAY

During each Wellness Week, Day 5 (typically Friday) is known as Get Fit Friday. On this day, a schoolwide event focusing on physical activity will be planned by the wellness coordinator. The Get Fit Friday activities are called TEAM Time activities (TEAM stands for Together Everyone Achieves More).

During Wellness Week 4, the TEAM Time activity planned for Get Fit Friday is called Mid Kids Lead. The wellness coordinator will teach several third and fourth grade students how to do the routine ahead of time so that they can help lead. Then the wellness coordinator and the selected students will lead the TEAM Time activity at the beginning of the school day. All students in the school will congregate outside or in the gym or multipurpose room so that they all can participate together. The activity includes a warm-up, a workout routine, and a cool-down.

In addition to supporting Mid Kids Lead, mention the TEAM Time activity as you discuss the video routine messages during the morning activity break.

## MORNING ACTIVITY BREAK

**DVD Routine**: It's the One

### Introduction

"We've been doing the It's the One video all week, so today we should be getting pretty good at it. I hope you can sing along as you do it. Try it. Trying hard means paying attention to what you are doing, but when you have done that a lot and you get really good, sometimes you just do it without even having to think about it. Let's see if we can do this routine easily."

### Video Routine

The DVD has five versions of the It's the One routine, one for each day of the week. It also has a special instructional version that teaches students how to do the routine.

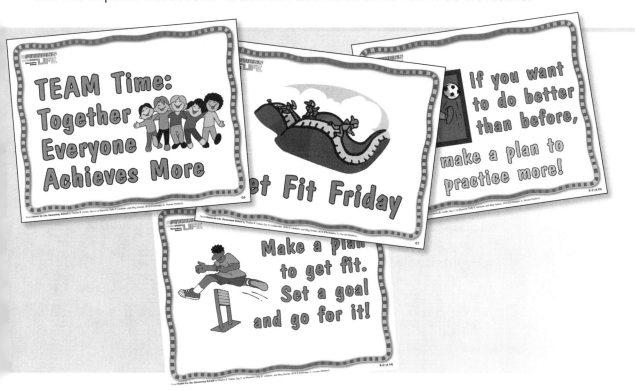

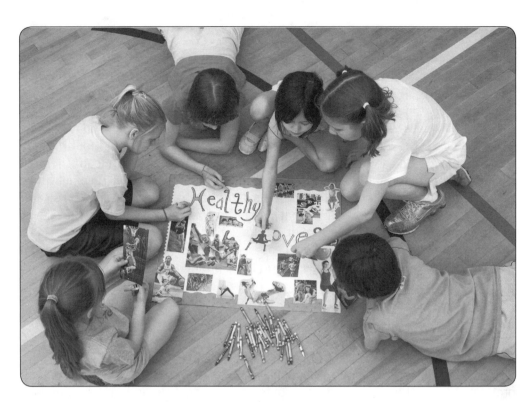

When you want to get better at something, start by creating a simple plan or picture to help you focus.

1. If the students have not done this week's routine before, play the instructional routine. If the PE teacher has already taught the routine to the students, or if they have already practiced the instructional routine with you, you can skip this step.
2. Play the Day 5 routine.

Each day the current version of the routine promotes a new and different message. Variations on the message play before the first routine, between routines, and after the last routine. For It's the One, the Day 5 message is "Plan to get better," and the three variations are as follows:

* If you want to get better, you need a plan; write down what you want to do, and say, "I can."

* If you want to do something better than before, make a plan to practice more and more.

* If you want to do something better, writing a plan is the first step. Maybe your plan is to practice, or maybe it's to try something new. Whatever your plan is, it can only start with you.

## Breathing

After finishing the routine, lead the class in breathing.

"Breathing deeply is important for our bodies, so we'll end every activity with a couple of deep breaths. Let's all breathe in deeply (count 1, 2), hold (count 1, 2), breathe out (count 1, 2), and hold (count 1, 2)." Repeat three times.

## Background Information

* Planning can help you focus on what you want to do.
* You can write a simple plan to help you get better; you could even draw a picture of you practicing or trying something new!
* When you want to try something new, part of your plan can be to find a friend who can help.
* Keeping your plan where you can see it reminds you to do it.
* Thinking of little steps to get to your goal really helps you get there.

## Discussion

* "Do you remember ever making a plan for something you wanted?"
* "Did you write it down or draw a picture to remind you?"
* "Is there something we'd like to get better at as a class? Let's make a plan." (To make a plan, identify the goal; identify two strategies for reaching the goal; choose a way to make a record if the strategies are being executed; and identify how to know when the goal is met.)

## Chant

Chanting is a great way to reinforce messages. If you've posted the corresponding sign, point to it, and tell the students that when you say the first phrase, they should respond by saying the second phrase. Make it fun!

Teacher: "If you want to do better than before . . ."

Students: ". . . make a plan to practice more!"

Practice several times until the students respond easily to your prompt.

> **teacher tip** • • •
> "Nice time" refers to taking a few minutes to allow and encourage students to compliment each other on their work. Starting with a stem such as "I'd like to compliment _____ because she did a great job of _____" teaches the students how to identify a particular action to compliment. If you honor this time, the students will, too.

## Closure

Closure provides an opportunity to focus one more time on the main message of the lesson by using compliments, reviewing messages, and making suggestions for doing activity at home.

### *Compliments*

"You're getting so good at the routine that you can almost do it without thinking about it. As a class, we are looking good!"

### *Take It Home*

"Is there something you'd like to make a plan about at home? Ask someone to help you write it down."

> **review** • • •
> "Do you feel excited when you make a plan about something? Do you find yourself thinking about it more and more? This week we did the It's the One routine. We've been talking about balancing how much we eat and how active we are and making plans about getting better."

WEEK **4** • DAY **5**

## AFTERNOON ACTIVITY BREAK

**Activity**: Birthday Lineup

Perform in the afternoon or at some other time during the day when the students need a physical activity break.

"Remember during last Wellness Week, we lined up in order of our shoe colors. We're going to line up in birthday order today. We could do it two ways, by the date—like the 4th—or by the month—like October. Let's do it by the month first. Think of your birthday. What month is it in?" Call out months starting with January and have children line up accordingly.

> **interdisciplinary • • •**
> This activity requires practice in sequencing as well as movement.

"Now that we are lined up, let's do our lineup routine. Let's clap once, jump two times, march three times, and run in place four times. Let's do it again."

Repeat the activity with the date. Ask, "What number is the date of your birthday? Raise your hand if it is on the first, second, third . . . So let's line up with the first here, then second . . . Let's do our lineup routine."

Pose questions about the data. How many children have birthdays in each month? Make an estimate first, then sort students by their birthday month and do a count. (You could also play Simon Says and have students get in groups by birth months.)

### Breathing

After finishing the activity, lead the class in breathing.

"Breathing deeply is important for our bodies, so we'll end every activity with a couple of deep breaths. Let's all breathe in deeply (count 1, 2), hold (count 1, 2), breathe out (count 1, 2), and hold (count 1, 2)." Repeat three times.

### Closure

"You are good listeners and thinkers. Thanks for showing such good body control. Birthdays are special days. It doesn't matter where you were in the line—your birthday is a special day for you. Today you worked as a team, and we lined up by birthday. I heard people helping each other to figure it out by giving suggestions. I heard other people say, 'OK,' 'Thanks,' and 'Right.'"

## ADDITIONAL ACTIVITIES

See appendix A for additional enriching and integrative outdoor activities. For more information, go to www.fitnessforlife.org.

WEEK 4 • DAY 5

# A P P E N D I X

# A

# Additional Activities

This appendix contains additional activities that can be used at any time for an activity break during the day or substituted for the afternoon activity break. The activities often combine simple practice of movement and an academic skill. They were intentionally chosen to be simple and basic. A few examples of activities in each category are provided to get you started and stimulate your thinking. You can adapt the ideas to match your own curriculum.

## Physical Activities

This section presents sample activities that can be done outdoors along with activities that relate to basic math skills, language arts skills, and art skills.

## Outdoor Activities

The activities below are simple and easy to do. They are performed outside rather than in the classroom. They will get everyone moving quickly and are easy to extend and adapt. These activities can be done anytime a break is needed, substituted for the afternoon physical activity break, or used as recess activities.

### Start and Stop

Using cones, milk jugs, rope, or something similar, create a boundary marking where the students can move around. Start by having students move around in the area and stopping on a signal. The signal can be a whistle, bell, or math problem; for instance, they stop when you call out a number larger than 5, an even number, a number less than 10, and so on.

Start with walking, and as good body control is demonstrated, move to galloping, skipping, jogging, and running.

### Basic Tag

Play Start and Stop first to ensure good body control. If students have good body control, introduce Tag.

In this game, the taggers want to tag non-taggers, and non-taggers want to avoid being tagged. Have something to identify taggers (a scarf, pinnie, wrist band, rag ball, or soft noodle piece to carry). Choose one-fourth of the students to be taggers and give each an identifying item. When a tagger tags someone, she gives that person the item and that person is the new tagger. Have the children practice gentle tagging and then discuss what is and is not appropriate.

Start with everyone walking. When good body control and rule following is evident, change to galloping, then skipping, then jogging.

### Follow the Leader

Played around the playground, it's most fun when everyone is following you all around the area, or in groups of about six with the children taking turns being the leader.

## Physical Activity and Mathematics

Presented here are a few ideas to help you combine short activities with basic math skills. These activities can be done instead of one of the afternoon physical activity breaks in the lesson plans, used anytime as a quick break, or used as a method of transitioning to a new area or activity.

## Counting Activities

Create a list of activities that everyone can do 10 times. Count in different formats whenever you do those movements. Do them often for a fitness break.

### Activity 1: Activity Counts

Have students count how many repetitions they do of specific exercises. Start with 10 repetitions.

- 10 claps
- 10 stretches—alternate stretching the right hand and the left hand up high (or perform any other stretch you choose)

Increase the number of repetitions to 20.

- 20 marches, jumps, and so on

### Activity 2: Counting Steps

Have students count their steps as they walk.

- To the door
- Around the classroom
- To the cafeteria
- To the playground
- Around the playground

### Activity 3: Counting Using Different Formats

Have students count in different ways as they do activities.

- Forward (1, 2, 3, 4, 5, 6, 7, 8, 9, 10)
- Backward (10, 9, 8, 7, 6, 5, 4, 3, 2, 1)
- Counting by 2s, by 5s, by 10s (2, 4, 6, 8 . . .)
- Counting just the odd or even numbers (1, 3, 5, 7 . . .)

### Activity 4: Classifying/Categorizing

Use a white board or newsprint and marker.

- List activities that make you breathe fast. List activities you can do breathing normally.
- Make a list of foods and a list of physical activities. Try to have the same number of physical activities as foods.

### Activity 5: Data Collection and Graphing

You will need 2×2 sticky notes for sticky-note graphing. In a line across the bottom of the board, write possible answers to questions. Give each child a sticky note to place in a column (one above the other) above his chosen answer. Have them walk all the way around the room (or do 20 jumping jacks, or run in place 20 times) before placing their sticky. When all notes are posted, look at the bar graph they created and discuss which choices were most popular, least popular, and so on. Possible questions include:

- How many of your steps does it take to go around your desk? Students should choose from one of the following categories: 1 to 5 steps, 6 to 10 steps, 11 to 15 steps, or 16 to 20 steps.
- What cereal do you like for breakfast?
- What is your favorite vegetable? Fruit? Sport?

# Physical Activity and Language Arts

Presented here are a few ideas to stimulate your thinking about combining short activities with language arts skills. These can be done instead of one of the afternoon physical activity breaks in the lesson plans, used anytime as a quick break, or used as a method of transitioning to a new area or activity.

## Movement Stories to Act Out

Ask students to act out the stories described below.

### A Good Healthy Day

Create a movement story about a good healthy day. As the story is told, have all the children act it out in mime. You can create the story yourself, use the story below, or have the children create the story as a group writing lesson.

It's time to wake up in the morning. Chris stretches, yawns, and then looks around and smiles. This is going to be a great day. To start off, Chris washes his face and hands and gets dressed. Then Chris walks quickly to the kitchen and helps get out the cereal, milk, and bananas. Chris drinks a glass of orange juice, eats the cereal and milk, puts the dishes in the dishwasher, and goes outside to shoot some baskets before it's time to go to school. Pat comes by, and Chris and Pat put on their helmets and ride to school together. In school, they take good drinks at the drinking fountain. They know that drinking water is good for them. In class, Pat and Chris like doing the La Raspa video routine. At lunch, they drink some milk and have an apple and grapes with their sandwiches. At recess, they run (do in place) and play. After school, they play catch outside and then come in and dance to some music. At dinner, Chris says, "Counting these green beans, I've had five fruits and veggies today (count on fingers): bananas, orange juice, apple, grapes, and green beans. And I've had five colors: white; orange, red, purple, green." Chris looks at a good book and then goes to bed.

### Hop on Pop

Read Dr. Seuss' *Hop on Pop*. Every time you say the word "hop," everyone does a little jump (using two feet) in place. Count the number of times the *Hop on Pop* story says "hop."

### *Using Prompts to Encourage Writing*

Ask each student to write a short story using the following prompts.

- Write a class story about someone trying something lots of times in order to get better.
- Write a class rhyme about why physical activity is important.
- Write a class rhyme about why making good food choices is important.
- Write a class instruction book about how to play a chosen game.

## Physical Activity and Art

Presented here are a few ideas for using art to promote physical activity. Have students draw pictures related to physical activity using the following prompts.

- Have the children draw illustrations to accompany the week's signs and talk about the activities they choose to include.

- Encourage children to draw a picture that shows a physical activity they like to do.
- Encourage children to make up a story to tell a partner about the activity in their picture.
- Have the children draw their favorite fruits. Create a poster with a rainbow. Have the children name fruits of each color and put them on the bars of the rainbow.

# Nutrition Activities

This section provides sample activities to support nutrition concepts. The MyPyramid.gov activities help identify and reinforce nutrition basics. The suggested books and stories about nutrition help stimulate discussion. Additional activities connect nutrition information with simple math skills.

## MyPyramid Activities

MyPyramid for Kids (available at www.mypyramid.gov) is an educational tool developed by the United States Department of Agriculture to help children learn about good health and nutrition. Additional nutrition activities for consideration include the following:

- MyPyramid Coloring Page for lower grade levels. Available at: www.mypyramid.gov/kids/index_print.html (This resource is also available on the DVD for grades K-2 in each Wellness Week's Worksheets folder.)
- MyPyramid worksheets. Available at: http://teamnutrition.usda.gov/kids-pyramid.html
- MyPyramid for Kids: A Closer Look. This downloadable educational tool helps children learn basic concepts in MyPyramid for Kids. Available at: http://teamnutrition.usda.gov/Resources/mypyramidcloselook.html

## Nutrition and Mathematics: Classifying and Categorizing

Use a chalk or white board or newsprint and marker to

- Classifying: Make a list of foods with nutrients (e.g., fruits, veggies, dairy, meat, legumes, and so on) and another list of those that have empty calories (candy, sodas, and so forth—no nutrients), and

- Categorizing: Make a list of foods and a list of physical activities. Try to have the same number of physical activities as foods.

## Nutrition and Language Arts

The following are books and stories that involve nutrition. Encourage students to read the stories on their own, or read the stories to them followed by a nutrition discussion. The book titles and descriptions are reproduced as presented on the Web site of the School Nutrition Association. For more information, go to www.schoolnutrition.org.

- *Belly Laughs* by Charles Keller. These 75 food jokes and illustrations are written especially for children.

- *A Book of Fruit* by Barbara Hirsch Lember. While most children recognize fruit in a bowl or in a supermarket, some have never seen fruit growing on a tree or a bush. This well-photographed book makes the connection between the fruit and where and how it grows before it arrives at the supermarket. Photos of single servings of fruit appear on pages opposite photos of where the fruit grows.

- *Milk From Cow to Carton* by Aliki. Aliki takes readers on a guided tour that begins with grazing cows, proceeds through milking and a trip to the dairy, and ends with some different foods made from milk.

- *The Vegetable Show* by Laura Krasny Brown. Watch vegetables do a little vaudeville in their attempt to dance and sing their way onto the plates and into the hearts of kids. Kids will truly be tempted by the delightful characters including the Tip-Top Tomato Twins and Bud the Spud.

- *The Victory Garden Vegetable Alphabet Book* by Jerry Pallotta and Bob Thomson. This book depicts a vegetable for each letter of the alphabet. The art and text help students to make important associations between vegetables and other familiar things in the environment.

- *Dinosaurs Alive and Well: A Guide to Good Health* by Laurie Krasny Brown and Marc Brown. Colorful and bright dinosaurs provide kids with a blueprint to good health. Nutrition, exercise, and fitness are some of the topics that are encountered.

- *Bread Is for Eating* by David and Phillis Gershator. Mamita explains how bread is created and sings, "El Pan Es Para Comer" ("Bread Is for Eating"). Music and lyrics in both Spanish and English are included.

- *What Am I? Looking Through Shapes at Apples and Grapes* by Diane and Leo Dillon. Invite children to guess each food described in a rhyme and shown through a hole on the right-hand page. Turn the page for the answer!

©2009 School Nutrition Association: *School Nutrition.*

## Resources

Listed here are sample Web sites that provide great information on nutrition, physical activity, physical education, and health. Most include content and fun activities to help students clarify and internalize basic information related to these concepts.

### Nutrition Web Sites

www.mypyramid.gov (MyPyramid, government)

www.squaremeals.org (nutrition, organization)

www.dole.com/superkids/ (nutrition, commercial)

www.choosykids.com/CK2/ (nutrition and activity, commercial)

### Physical Activity Web Sites

www.fitness.gov (President's Council, government)

www.davidkatzmd.com/abcforfitness.aspx (fitness)

www.activeacademics.org (activity and academics, organization)

www.circusfit.com (circus fitness and skills, commercial)

## Physical Education Web Sites

www.pecentral.org (physical education, organization)

www.aahperd.org/naspe/ (physical education, organization)

www.ncpe4me.com/energizers.html (physical education, organization)

## Health Web Sites

www.preventioninstitute.org (university, organization)

www.aafp.org/online/en/home/clinical/publichealth/aim/aimschoolprgm/teacher.html (public health, organization)

# APPENDIX

## B

# NASPE and Other Standards

A variety of educational standards were consulted prior to preparing the materials in this guide. Physical education and nutrition standards were the primary sources for the lesson plans; however, many other standards were consulted as well. The authors felt that it was important to integrate wellness concepts (nutrition and physical activity) with concepts and standards from other subject matter areas. In this appendix, selected standards from many areas of study are listed. Only standards that related to the content of the lessons were used. Web addresses for more complete descriptions of standards are provided.

## Physical Education Standards for Grades K-2

Standards and performance outcomes adapted from: NASPE. (2004). *Moving into the future: National standards for physical education* (2nd ed.). Reston, VA: Author.

National standards for physical education were developed by the National Association for Sport and Physical Education (NASPE). There are six major standards. Within each of the six standards, there are selected performance outcomes. A list of performance outcomes is included below (by a number and a letter). The numbers and letters are included in the lesson plans in this book (e.g., 1A refers to the *motor skills and movement patterns* standard and to the *performs simple dance steps* outcome).

### Standard 1: Motor Skills and Movement Patterns

Children are active and enjoy learning and mastering new skills. Children achieve mature forms of movement patterns including more mature patterns using various body parts.

- 1A: Performs simple dance steps
- 1B: Demonstrates clear contrast between fast and slow movements—keeping tempo
- 1C: Demonstrates a smooth transition between locomotor skills in time to music
- 1D: Discovers how to balance on different body parts
- 1E: Performs more mature movement patterns using various body parts
- 1F: Enjoys learning new activities and skills

### Standard 2: Movement Concepts, Principles, Strategies, and Tactics Applied to Learning and Performance

Children mature in cognitive abilities associated with movement. They learn to apply concepts to movements and to identify correct form in movement performances.

- 2A: Identifies body planes (front, back, side)
- 2B: Identifies various body parts (knee, foot, arm, palm)
- 2C: States short-term effects of physical activity on heart and lungs
- 2D: Explains that appropriate practice improves performance
- 2E: Uses knowledge in movement situations

## Standard 3: Participates Regularly in Physical Activity

Children participate for pleasure and have fun while being active. They perform locomotor and non-locomotor activities and use them during free time. They recognize the temporary and lasting effects of activity on the body and choose to perform activities that benefit health.

- 3A: Engages in moderate to vigorous physical activity on an intermittent basis
- 3B: Engages in a variety of locomotor activities (hopping, walking, jumping)
- 3C: Has fun while being active
- 3D: Learns locomotor and non-locomotor activities, and uses them in free time
- 3E: Knows several health benefits of physical activity

## Standard 4: Achieves and Maintains Health-Enhancing Physical Fitness

Children engage in activities that enhance health-related fitness and enjoy it. They recognize factors associated with moderate to vigorous activity (e.g., sweating, fast heart rate, heavy breathing). Students have basic knowledge about and understand the five parts of health-related fitness.

- 4A: Demonstrates sufficient muscular strength to be able to bear body weight
- 4B: Engages in a series of locomotor activities (timed segments of hopping, walking, and so on) without easily tiring
- 4C: Recognizes physical responses to activity associated with fitness
- 4D: Participates in a variety of games that increase breathing and heart rate
- 4E: Sustains activity for increasingly longer periods of time while participating in various activities in physical education
- 4F: Recognizes that health-related physical fitness consists of several different parts

## Standard 5: Exhibits Responsible Personal and Social Behavior and Respect for Others in Activity

Children discover that playing with friends makes activities fun. They know safe practices and know how to apply rules. They use successful interpersonal communication during group activity. They appreciate cooperation in learning skills and cooperate, share, and work together to solve problems or meet a challenge.

- 5A: Practices specific skills as assigned until the teacher signals the end of practice
- 5B: Follows directions given to the class for an all-class activity
- 5C: Shows compassion for others by helping them
- 5D: Works in diverse group settings without interfering with others
- 5E: Enjoys working alone and in groups while exploring movement tasks
- 5F: Accepts all playmates without regard to personal differences (e.g., ethnicity, gender, disability)
- 5G: Displays consideration of others while participating
- 5H: Demonstrates the elements of socially acceptable conflict resolution during class activity
- 5I: Shares and works well with other children in activity settings

## Standard 6: Values Physical Activity for Health, Enjoyment, Challenge, Self-Expression, and Social Interaction

Children are active and enjoy participating. They meet challenges of new movements and skills. They feel joy when they achieve competence and begin to function as members of a group and use cooperation in activity.

- 6A: Exhibits both verbal and nonverbal indicators of enjoyment
- 6B: Willingly tries new movements and skills

- 6C: Continues to participate when not successful on the first try
- 6D: Identifies several activities that are enjoyable
- 6E: Expresses personal feelings on progress while learning a new skill
- 6F: Enjoys activity involvement and achieving motor skills
- 6G: Functions well with other children in group activities

# Selected Mathematics Standards for Grades K-2

National Council of Teachers of Mathematics http://standards.nctm.org/document/appendix/meas.htm

The selected standards listed below were considered in developing lessons for this book.

### Numbers and Operations

- Count with understanding.
- Understand relative position and magnitude of ordinal and cardinal numbers.
- Connect number words and numerals.

### Algebra

- Sort, classify, and order objects by size, number, and other qualities.
- Recognize, describe, and extend sequences and translate from one representation to another.
- Analyze how both repeating and growing patterns are generated.
- Model situations that involve addition and subtraction of whole numbers using objects, pictures, and symbols.

### Measurement

- Understand how to measure using non-standard and standard units.
- Select an appropriate unit and tool for the attribute being measured.
- Use repetition of a single unit to measure something larger than the unit; for instance, measuring the length of a room with a single meterstick.

- Develop common referents for measures to make comparisons and estimates.

### Data Analysis and Probability

- Pose questions and gather data about the self and surroundings.
- Sort and classify objects according to their attributes and organize data about the objects.
- Represent data using concrete objects, pictures, and graphs.
- Describe parts of the data and the set of data as a whole to determine what the data show.

# Science Standards for Grades K-4

National Science Education Standards. Center for Science, Mathematics, and Engineering Education. Selected from www.educationworld.com/standards/national/science/k_4.shtml

The selected standards listed below were considered in developing lessons for this book.

### Science as Inquiry

- Abilities necessary to do scientific inquiry
- Understanding about scientific inquiry

### Physical Science

- Properties of objects and materials
- Position and motion of objects

### Life Science

- Characteristics of organisms
- Organisms and environments

### Earth and Space Science

- Properties of earth materials

### Science and Technology

- Understanding about science and technology
- Abilities to distinguish between natural objects and objects made by humans

### Personal and Social Perspectives

- Personal health
- Characteristics and changes in populations
- Changes in environments
- Science and technology in local challenges

*History of Nature and Science*

- Science as a human endeavor

# Language Arts Standards for Grades K-12

Selected from www.ncte.org/standards

The selected standards listed below were considered in developing lessons for this book.

- Students adjust their use of spoken, written, and visual language (e.g., conventions, style, vocabulary) to communicate effectively with a variety of audiences and for different purposes.

- Students employ a wide range of strategies as they write and use different writing process elements appropriately to communicate with different audiences for a variety of purposes.

- Students apply knowledge of language structure, language conventions (e.g., spelling and punctuation), media techniques, figurative language, and genre to create, critique, and discuss print and non-print texts.

- Students conduct research on issues and interests by generating ideas and questions, and by posing problems. They gather, evaluate, and synthesize data from a variety of sources (e.g., print and non-print texts, artifacts, people) to communicate their discoveries in ways that suit their purpose and audience.

- Students use a variety of technological and information resources (e.g., libraries, databases, computer networks, video) to gather and synthesize information and to create and communicate knowledge.

- Students use spoken, written, and visual language to accomplish their own purposes (e.g., for learning, enjoyment, persuasion, and the exchange of information).

# Civics Standards for Grades K-4

National Council for the Social Studies. Selected from www.educationworld.com/standards/national/soc_sci/civics/k_4.shtml

The selected standards listed here were considered in developing lessons for this book.

## What Is Government?

- What are the purposes of rules and laws?
- How can you evaluate rules and laws?

## Values and Principles of Democracy

- Why is it important for Americans to share certain values, principles, and beliefs?
- What are the benefits of diversity in the United States?
- How should conflicts about diversity be prevented or managed?
- How can people work together to promote the values and principles of American democracy?

## Roles of the Citizen

- What are important responsibilities of Americans?
- What dispositions or traits of character are important to the preservation and improvement of American democracy?

# Geography Standards for Grades K-12

Selected from www.educationworld.com/standards/national/soc_sci/geography/k_12.shtml

The selected standard listed below was considered in developing lessons for this book.

## The World in Spatial Terms

- Understand how to use maps and other geographic representations, tools, and technologies to acquire, process, and report information from a spatial perspective.

# U.S. History Standards for Grades K-4

National Center for History in the Schools. Selected from www.educationworld.com/standards/national/soc_sci/us_history/k_4.shtml

The selected standards listed below were considered in developing lessons for this book.

## Living and Working Together in Families and Communities

- Understand family life now and in the past, and family life in various places long ago.

### The History of the United States: Democratic Principles and Values

- Understand how democratic values came to be, and how they have been exemplified by people, events, and symbols.
- Understand the folklore and other cultural contributions from various regions of the United States, and how they helped to form a national heritage.

### The History of Peoples of Many Cultures

- Understands selected attributes and historical developments of societies in Africa, the Americas, Asia, and Europe.

# REFERENCES AND SUGGESTED RESOURCES

Corbin, C.B., & Pangrazi, R.P. (2001). Toward a uniform definition of wellness: A commentary. *President's Council on Physical Fitness and Sports Research Digest, 3*(15), 1-8. Available at www.fitness.gov/publications/digests/pcpfs_research_digs.html.

Graham, G. (2008). *Teaching children physical education* (3rd ed.). Champaign, IL: Human Kinetics.

Hillman, C.H., Buck, S.M., Themanson, J.R., Pontifex, M.B., & Castelli, D. (2009a). Aerobic fitness and cognitive development: Event-related brain potential and task performance indices of executive control in preadolescent children. *Developmental Psychology, 45*, 114-129.

Hillman, C.H., Pontifex, M.B., Raine, L.B., Castelli, D.M., Hall, E.E., & Kramer, A.F. (2009b). The effect of acute treadmill walking on cognitive control and academic achievement in preadolescent children. *Neuroscience, 159*, 1044-1054.

Le Masurier, G.C., & Corbin, C.B. (2006). Top 10 reasons for quality physical education. *Journal of Physical Education, Recreation and Dance, 77*(6), 44-53.

National Association for Sport and Physical Education (NASPE). (2004). *Moving into the future: National standards for physical education* (2nd ed.). Reston, VA: Author.

Ogden, C.L., Carroll, M.D., & Flegal, K.M. (2008). High body mass index for age among US children and adolescents, 2003-2006. *Journal of the American Medical Association, 299*(20), 2401-2405.

Ratey, J.J. (2008). *SPARK: The revolutionary new science of exercise and the brain.* New York: Little, Brown.

Smith, N.J., & Lounsbery, M. (2009). Promoting physical education: The link to academic achievement. *Journal of Physical Education, Recreation and Dance, 80*(1), 39-43.

United States Department of Health and Human Services (USDHHS). (2008). 2008 physical activity guidelines for Americans: Be active, healthy, and happy. Washington, DC: Author. www.health.gov/paguidelines/guidelines/default.aspx.

United States Department of Health and Human Services (USDHHS), & U.S. Department of Agriculture (USDA). (2005). *Dietary guidelines for Americans, 2005* (6th ed.). Washington, DC: U.S. Government Printing Office. Available at: www.health.gov/DietaryGuidelines/dga2005/document/default.htm.

World Health Organization (WHO). (1947). Constitution of the World Health Organization. *Chronicle of the World Health Organization, 1*, 29-43.

# ABOUT THE AUTHORS

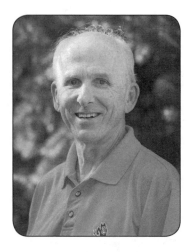

**Charles B. "Chuck" Corbin, PhD,** is currently professor emeritus in the department of exercise and wellness at Arizona State University. He has published more than 200 journal articles and is the senior author of, sole author of, contributor to, or editor of more than 80 books, including the 5th edition of *Fitness for Life* (winner of the TAA's Texty Award), the 14th edition of *Concepts of Physical Fitness* (winner of the TAA's McGuffey Award), and the 7th edition of *Concepts of Fitness and Wellness*. His books are the most widely adopted high school and college texts in fitness and wellness. Dr. Corbin is internationally recognized as an expert in physical activity, health and wellness promotion, and youth physical fitness. He has presented keynote addresses at more than 40 state AHPERD conventions, made major addresses in more than 15 countries, and presented numerous named lectures (Cureton, ACSM; Hanna, Sargent, and Distinguished Scholar, NAKPEHE; Prince Phillip, British PEA; and Weiss and Alliance Scholar, AAHPERD). He is past president and fellow of AAKPE, fellow in the NASHPERDP, an ACSM fellow, and a lifetime member of AAHPERD. Among his awards are the Healthy American Fitness Leaders Award (President's Council on Physical Fitness and Sports—PCPFS, National Jaycees), AAHPERD Honor Award, Physical Fitness Council Honor Award, the COPEC Hanson Award, and the Distinguished Service Award of the PCPFS. Dr. Corbin was named the Alliance Scholar by AAHPERD and the Distinguished Scholar of NAKPEHE. He is a member of the Fitnessgram Advisory Board and was the first chair of the science board of the PCPFS and the NASPE Hall of Fame. In 2009 Dr. Corbin was chosen for the Gulick Award, the highest award of AAHPERD.

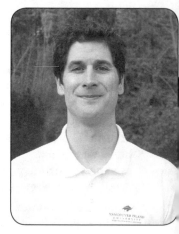

**Guy Le Masurier, PhD,** is a professor of physical education at Vancouver Island University, where he teaches courses in pedagogy, research methods, and nutrition for health and sport. Dr. Le Masurier is coauthor of the award-winning book *Fitness for Life: Middle School* (winner of the TAA's Texty Award) and has edited and contributed to several books, including the 5th edition of *Fitness for Life* and the *Physical Best Activity Guide*. He has published numerous articles related to youth physical activity and physical education and served as a coauthor on the *NASPE Physical Activity Guidelines for Children*. Dr. Le Masurier has delivered over 30 research and professional presentations at national and regional meetings and currently serves as the Epidemiology section editor for *Research Quarterly for Exercise and Sport* as well as the Health Foundations section editor for the *International Journal of Physical Education*. Dr. Le Masurier is the creator of the Walk Everyday Live Longer (WELL) program, a pedometer-based physical activity program used by the Arizona Department of Health Services. Dr. Le Masurier is a member of AAHPERD, NASPE, and ACSM. He lives with his wife on Protection Island in British Columbia, where they serve their community as volunteer firefighters. Guy is thankful for his morning kayak commutes.

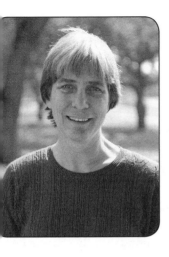

**Dolly D. Lambdin, EdD,** is a senior lecturer in the department of kinesiology and health education at the University of Texas at Austin, where she teaches undergraduate courses in children's movement and methods of teaching as well as graduate courses in analysis of teaching and technology application in physical education.

Dr. Lambdin taught elementary physical education in public and private schools for 16 years and taught preservice teachers for 33 years at the university level. During much of that time, she taught simultaneously at both levels, a situation that required her to spend part of each day meeting the teaching and research demands of academia while tackling the daily adventure of teaching 5- to 14-year-olds. In addition, she has supervised over 100 student teachers, and as a result has been able to visit classes and learn from scores of wonderful cooperating teachers in the schools.

Dr. Lambdin has served as the president of NASPE (2004-05) and on the NASPE board of directors for two three-year terms. She has also served on numerous local, state, and national committees, including the writing teams for the Texas Essential Knowledge and Skills in Physical Education, the NASPE Beginning Teacher Standards, the Texas Beginning Teacher Standards, and the NASPE Appropriate Practices Revision. Dr. Lambdin has been honored as the Texas AHPERD Outstanding College and University Physical Educator of the Year.

**Meg Greiner, MEd,** is a national board-certified elementary physical education teacher at Independence Elementary School in Independence, Oregon. She has been teaching elementary physical education for 21 years and regularly receives student teachers and practicum students

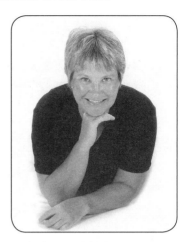

into her setting. Meg has received numerous national awards and accolades for her innovative physical education program and the development of TEAM Time, including the 2005 NASPE National Elementary Physical Education Teacher of the Year, 2005 *USA Today* All-USA Teacher Team, and the 2006 Disney Outstanding Specialist Teacher of the Year. Meg is currently working with NASPE as a Head Start Body Start trainer of trainers, serving on the AAHPERD Physical Best Committee, and presenting NASPE Pipeline Workshops all over the United States. She has served on the NASPE Council of Physical Education for Children and on the public relations committee. She has served as the physical education president for both Oregon and Northwest District AHPERDs. She also has served Oregon AHPERD in many capacities and has received the OAHPERD Honor Award.

# DVD USER INSTRUCTIONS

The DVD-ROM contains videos and resources to use with the **Fitness for Life: Elementary School** classroom lesson plans. This section provides the technical details for accessing the contents of the disc. For information about how to use the videos and resources in class, see "Using the DVD" on page 16.

## Videos

When you insert the disc in a DVD player, the TV screen displays a Main Menu of your grade's activity routines for Wellness Weeks 1, 2, 3, and 4. Select the routine for the current week, and you'll see a submenu that lets you play the instructional routine (which teaches the movements to your students) or one of the daily activity routines (which students follow and perform).

## Resources

The resources can be viewed only on a computer with a DVD-ROM drive. To access the resources, follow the instructions for Microsoft Windows® or Macintosh® computers.

### *Microsoft Windows*

1. Place the DVD in the DVD-ROM drive of your computer.
2. Double-click on the "My Computer" icon from your desktop.
3. Right-click on the DVD-ROM drive and select the "Open" option from the pop-up menu.
4. Open the Resources folder and then the General folder or one of the Wellness Week folders to find the desired resource.
5. Select the file you want to view and print.

### *Macintosh*

1. Place the DVD in the DVD-ROM drive of your computer.
2. Double-click on the DVD icon on your desktop.
3. Open the Resources folder and then the General folder or one of the Wellness Week folders to find the desired resource.
4. Select the file that you want to view and print.

You will need Adobe® Reader® to view the PDF files.